the internal family systems workbook

Also by Dr Richard C. Schwartz, PhD

No Bad Parts: Healing Trauma and Restoring Wholeness with the Internal Family Systems Model

You Are the One You've Been Waiting For: Applying Internal Family Systems to Intimate Relationships

Introduction to Internal Family Systems, 2nd edition

Internal Family Systems Therapy, 2nd edition (with Martha Sweezy)

Family Therapy: Concepts and Methods, 7th edition (with Michael P. Nichols)

The Mosaic Mind: Empowering the Tormented Selves of Child Abuse Survivors (with Regina A. Goulding)

Metaframeworks: Transcending the Models of Family Therapy (with Douglas C. Breunlin)

Handbook of Family Therapy Training and Supervision (with Howard A. Liddle and Douglas C. Breunlin)

Many Minds, One Self: Evidence for a Radical Shift in Paradigm (with Robert Falconer)

the internal family systems workbook

a guide to discover your self
and heal your parts

Dr RICHARD C. SCHWARTZ

Vermilion
LONDON

Vermilion, an imprint of Ebury Publishing
One Embassy Gardens, 8 Viaduct Gardens,
Nine Elms, London SW11 7BW

Vermilion is part of the Penguin Random House group of companies
whose addresses can be found at global.penguinrandomhouse.com

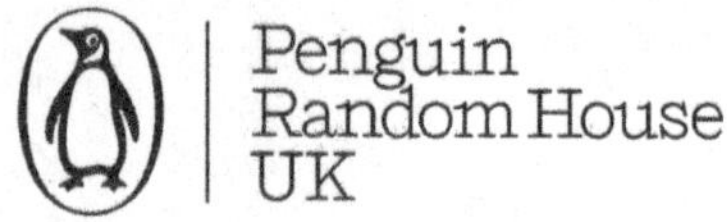

First published in Great Britain by Vermilion in 2024
First published in the United States of America by Sounds True in 2024

www.penguin.co.uk

A CIP catalogue record for this book is available from the British Library

ISBN 9781785045721

Printed and bound in Great Britain by Clays Ltd, Elcograf S.p.A.

The authorised representative in the EEA is Penguin Random House Ireland, Morrison Chambers, 32 Nassau Street, Dublin D02 YH68

contents

part two appreciating your overworked managers

part three befriending your activated firefighters

part four embracing your burdened exiles

part five accessing your unlimited self-leadership

introduction to IFS

I contain multitudes.

Walt Whitman

Welcome! I'm so glad you had the curiosity and courage to pick up this workbook. I want to start by welcoming you and all your parts on this internal journey of Self-discovery and healing. Internal Family Systems (IFS) is a dynamic way to connect with your own Self-energy, heal your parts, and engage the world with greater compassion.

You probably picked up this book for a reason. Maybe a part of you is longing to be seen and understood on a deeper level. Perhaps you hope to heal from past wounds that just won't seem to go away. Part of you may be desiring a spiritual connection or maybe you're just wanting simple strategies to live with more inner peace and harmony.

Another part of you may be looking for ways to be more courageous in your personal or professional relationships. Maybe a part of you is curious to see what the IFS hype is all about. You might even have a skeptical part that doesn't believe anything will help or change your current situation.

It's possible that some, if not all, of the above are true. That's because we all have a system of parts inside us, and those parts are working to help us, but sometimes they lead us astray, and they require us to dig deep to find out what those parts need from us.

Perhaps you've found yourself in a dilemma where one part of you says, "Do it," and another part of you says, "Don't you dare!" Or maybe you find yourself doing or saying something that you know will make a situation worse, but you can't stop yourself. Why do you do this? These aren't just random thoughts or impulses. If you focus on the impulse—ask questions of it—you'd learn that it's much more than that. It's actually a part simply trying to protect another part(s) of you.

IFS offers a way to befriend and embrace your entire inner system of parts. We can call this "parts work." In this workbook, you'll be doing your own parts work. A basic assumption of IFS is that everyone has a Self. This Self we refer to is similar to what others have described as the higher self or the soul. It is the core of you that exudes what we call the 8 Cs: Calm, Clarity, Confidence, Curiosity, Connectedness, Creativity, Compassion, and Courage. This Self cannot be damaged and has the ability to heal your parts. In addition to Self, you have an inner system, or your family of parts. These parts are often younger parts of you that developed strategies early in life in order to keep you protected, and often no longer serve you. When you learn to access the Self through this work, you will find that you have the profound ability to lead with Self rather than letting your parts run the show.

It may feel sometimes like some parts of you are trying to sabotage or harm you, but as you get deeper into the work, you will find that even your seemingly destructive parts are actually trying to help you. In IFS, all parts are welcome.

There are no bad parts.

Parts are well intentioned even when they take on extreme roles that end up doing more harm than good. Parts are like inner children thrust into extreme roles that are beyond their capacity to manage or cope. Even as you age, they get stuck in the age that the trauma took place, and from there, they take on burdens and responsibilities for protecting you, the family, or the system that are completely out of their scope. A lot of them are like parentified inner children—inner children who have taken on the roles of parents, even though they don't have the experience or maturity for these responsibilities—who need to be loved and finally relieved of these roles. When we learn to see them this way, to listen to their stories, we can become compassionate, offering comfort to them and connection with Self.

As you learn to access your Self-energy, you will be able to connect with your parts, and extend healing to them so that your parts can more consciously choose how to help you navigate life instead of overwhelming or burdening you. It is possible to live with your parts harmoniously. This simple yet transformative approach has not only become a proven model of therapy, it is a way of life.

The IFS practices you will learn in this workbook can help you:

- Stay calm when your parts are activated
- Gain clarity in your life purpose
- Keep your heart open
- Be more vulnerable
- Develop more Self-confidence
- Face your fears with courage
- Feel more integrated with your body, mind, and soul
- Overcome anxiety
- Heal from past wounds and trauma
- Extend more compassion toward yourself and others

Developing and sharing IFS with individuals and communities around the world has been my life's work for the last forty years. It's been a joy and a privilege to witness the spread of IFS, and to see the ways it is bringing healing and hope to so many. I am beyond thrilled to share these life-changing practices with you.

I am convinced that the IFS model has the ability to heal because I've seen it for myself, and I've heard from people all over the world who have used it to discover their Self, heal from trauma, and become more compassionate people. It has worked for me and countless others. I trust it can work for you, too. Packed with over fifty interactive exercises and meditations (visit soundstrue.com/the-ifs-workbook-bonus for guided audio meditations—watch for the QR code throughout the book), this workbook is uniquely designed to help you and your parts find harmony, inner healing, and hope.

Overview of Your Inner System

Your internal system consists of your Self, parts thrust into the roles of hardworking protectors called *managers* or *firefighters*, and your most vulnerable parts (that get hurt and then locked away inside) called *exiles*. Protector parts want to keep you safe. They'll do anything to protect you from pain, shame, and emotional overwhelm. Manager parts (like perfectionistic parts or inner critics) work preemptively to keep you out of your body and away from uncomfortable emotions by controlling and ordering your life, while firefighters (like confrontational or overindulging parts) are reactive to painful emotions or situations that activate you. Firefighters want to rescue you from uncomfortable feelings or unsafe people by fighting, comforting, soothing, or numbing. The exiles are the vulnerable, young parts of you that carry wounds and emotional burdens. They are often locked away inside for fear they'll be hurt again, or their pain would be too much for you. Exiles hold your deepest sadness, disappointment, and sorrow, so it can take time to gain their trust and heal them.

You will have a chance to explore all these parts in the pages ahead and establish deep connections between your Self and all of your parts.

The Power of IFS

There are four goals of IFS that you will have the opportunity to explore in this workbook:

1. The first is the liberation of parts from extreme roles. By showing compassion to your parts, they are able to transform. An overworked part can learn to relax and enjoy life. An overly critical part can offer helpful advice rather than scathing critique.

2. Secondly, IFS helps parts know they don't have to run everything. Things go better when they trust Self. Parts need to learn that you aren't a little kid anymore. They can trust Self to lead.

3. Third, IFS helps parts to know each other and live more harmoniously. Conflicting parts can learn to appreciate what other parts bring and you can experience more wholeness and peace inside.

4. Lastly, IFS can help bring more Self-leadership to your external world. Self-leadership is the ability to connect with your Self and parts so you can live from a place of courage, compassion, and curiosity. When you have compassion for your own parts, you're able to extend more compassion outwardly to your family, friends, and community.

How to Use This Workbook

This workbook will help you apply these transformative tools to your own life. I invite you to explore the parts that make up your internal system and extend compassion to each part of your Self as you make progress on your unique healing journey. Though IFS is simple to learn, it can take a lifetime to master. Even those who have been practicing for forty years continue to work with their parts and gain new insights, so I encourage you to take it slow, and be patient with yourself as the wisdom of your Self reveals itself to you and you make new discoveries about your parts. You'll be surprised at what you find.

Remember, even a small amount of parts work can make a big difference in your well-being.

The exercises in the workbook build on each other, so make sure you start with Part One before moving on to Parts Two through Five. You can repeat exercises and go back to exercises to build your skill and confidence. There are guided meditations throughout the workbook to help you practice going inside and connecting with your parts.

You may connect with a few parts or many. There is no right number of parts. Some parts may indicate the names they prefer, or you may only become aware of an impulse, feeling, or image. Don't worry about doing this perfectly. If you're growing in curiosity and compassion toward your parts, then you're doing it right.

You can decide the pace and depth you want to go. If you are new to the IFS model, these practices might take some adjustment. Take your time. You may have parts that are not ready for an exercise. That's okay. Listen to your parts and only proceed when you have their consent. You may have parts that want to rush through the workbook or distract you from it. Find the rhythm that works for you.

For many, IFS is a daily practice of listening to, connecting with, and feeling compassion for parts, leading to a deep and soulful connection. You may even choose to utilize the meditations and exercises as a form of spiritual practice, or connect them with your existing spiritual practices. Whether you see them as tools for Self-discovery or something more mystical, this is an embodied, experiential model that works best when it is practiced regularly in the course of your everyday life.

Going Inside

Parts work is, in general, an opportunity to go within. Throughout the workbook, however, you will come across "Going Inside" prompts. These are further opportunities within exercises to stop, look inward, and practice any given exercise more deeply. We're used to reading books to accumulate knowledge and build up our mental acumen, but this workbook is designed to be experiential, so you are invited to go inside and actually try this stuff out. Some of these exercises might seem foreign to you at first, but my hope is that you will find them useful for your journey, and they will encourage you to meet your parts with maximum compassion and curiosity.

IFS changes lives. It is an evidence-based approach with a proven track record to bring more healing, Self-energy, and hope to the world. Now it is your turn to experience this transformative tool for yourself. This might be the most important journey you ever take. You've got this!

Warmly,

Dick Schwartz

setting your intention

As you embark on this journey of Self-discovery, I invite you to set an intention. Think about what you hope to get from this process (for example, Self-awareness, healing, integration, spiritual connectivity, Self-leadership, compassion for Self and others, etc.).

Fill in your intention and sign your name to commit to the journey:

This workbook belongs to: ______________________________

My intention for going on this IFS journey is:

____

____

____

____

____

____

____

____

In the IFS model, consent and contracting are very important. You and you alone decide the pace and depth you want to go. All exercises and meditations are optional. By signing below, you agree that you are taking responsibility for what feels best for your inner system.

I understand that this workbook is intended to support my own exploration of my inner system. It is not a replacement for therapy.

I hereby consent and commit to this journey of personal exploration and growth.

x ______________________________ **date:** ______________________________

IFS Self-assessment

To begin your journey, take a few moments to fill out this IFS Self-assessment. This will help you assess what areas you may find most useful to focus on in your healing IFS journey.

Answer as honestly as you can. Check the boxes that are generally true for you (check all that apply):

- ❍ I often feel overwhelmed by my emotions
- ❍ I have trouble accessing my emotions
- ❍ I have difficulty communicating my emotions to loved ones
- ❍ I often work to the point of burnout
- ❍ I have trouble setting healthy boundaries with others
- ❍ I feel a lot of rage inside
- ❍ It's hard for me to speak up
- ❍ I sometimes don't know why I make certain choices
- ❍ I often regret things I've said to others or actions I've taken

- ❍ I fear embarrassing myself in public
- ❍ I wish I could control my anger
- ❍ Sometimes I spiral into depression
- ❍ Sometimes I get panic attacks
- ❍ I think I might have PTSD
- ❍ I have childhood wounds that still need healing
- ❍ I have unresolved conflict in some of my relationships
- ❍ I am easily triggered by things people say
- ❍ I wish I could silence my inner critic
- ❍ I say "yes" when I really want to say "no"
- ❍ Sometimes I feel like there are parts of me in conflict with each other
- ❍ I would like more harmony and peace inside
- ❍ I have a lot of negative self-talk
- ❍ I struggle to have compassion for people I disagree with
- ❍ I'm hard on myself when I make mistakes
- ❍ I have bouts of anxiety
- ❍ I would like to be more courageous
- ❍ I want to have more curiosity with people I don't understand
- ❍ I avoid conflict
- ❍ I wish I wasn't so passive
- ❍ I feel burdened by all the unrest in the world
- ❍ I would like to learn more about how my family and culture(s) impacts me today
- ❍ I have behaviors or habits I would like to change
- ❍ I desire to be a more confident leader

As you read this list and spent time with each statement, how did you feel? Were there particular statements that resonated strongly with you? Did many resonate with you, or just a few? These statements are meant to describe how a particular part, or parts of you, may impact your thoughts, emotions, or actions. As you move through this workbook, try to have compassion for these parts—even the ones you would like to shift. They are part of you for a reason. They are trying to help you. Tune in to them and try to understand them a bit more. Whether you checked a few boxes or a lot, this workbook will be a useful tool for your Self-discovery.

IFS Tip

IFS has been used extensively as a therapeutic tool by mental health professionals. This workbook takes some of the practices that are used in a therapeutic setting and presents them in a form for use by individuals. If at any time, as you work through this workbook, you feel overwhelmed, please reach out for support to a friend or mental health professional. If you do not have existing resources available, resources for support are listed at the back of this book.

an intro meditation

Throughout the workbook, there will be guided meditations to connect with your Self and parts. This practice is designed to help your parts know they aren't alone and that you are here to support them on this journey. Unlike some traditional meditation practices where the goal can be to quiet the mind, IFS meditations are opportunities to "tune in" to the mind and body. Our goal is to slow down input from the outside world and deeply listen to our internal systems. These messages may come in the form of colors, shapes, emotions, feelings in the body, or words or phrases. The messages are all welcome during an IFS meditation—they are from our parts. To begin, find a comfortable chair to sit on and sit upright, with your back straight and your mind alert. An audio recording of this practice is available at:

soundstrue.com/the-ifs-workbook-bonus

Take a couple of deep breaths.

Notice your body in your chair.

As you breathe deeply, scan your body for any points of pressure, congestion, stiffness, pain, or anything in or around your body that doesn't feel like you exactly. You can scan your mind also. Look for places of agitation in your mind, like dullness, fogginess, or anything that doesn't feel quite like you. These places are where we find our parts.

Then go ahead and begin to gently focus on that place in your body or in your mind while you continue to breathe deeply.

As you notice it, see if you can help it notice you. Help it notice it is not alone.

If it's possible, extend a loving energy or kindness to that place in your body or mind. You may find that other parts don't like this one and don't want you to show it love. If that's true, then don't try to force it and instead get to know the reasons the others don't like it.

At this point there might be something that it wants you to know. This is fine, but the main purpose of this meditation is to really let the part that is presenting know that they're not alone.

You can do that by extending a loving energy to it, offering some comforting words, or even breathing into it. Try one or all of those with this place in your mind or body.

The purpose of this practice is to help these parts know they're not alone, that they're loved, and that they can relax.

They're not alone because you're there, too. They can trust you. Some of them, as you extend the loving energy, comforting words, or breath, may sense an immediate relaxing. You may notice such a shift in your body or mind. Others won't shift, which is fine. It just means that they need more attention before they can relax. They may have more that they want you to hear or know.

As you stay with one part, and it doesn't relax, you can make an appointment to talk with it later and move on to another.

When you get to the other, you can extend that loving energy, comforting word, or breath, until you notice a shift.

When a part does relax, you'll notice a little more space in your body or mind, a little more openness.

When the time feels right, you can shift focus from your body and mind and return to the outside by opening your eyes and returning to the room you're in.

part one

getting to know your self & parts

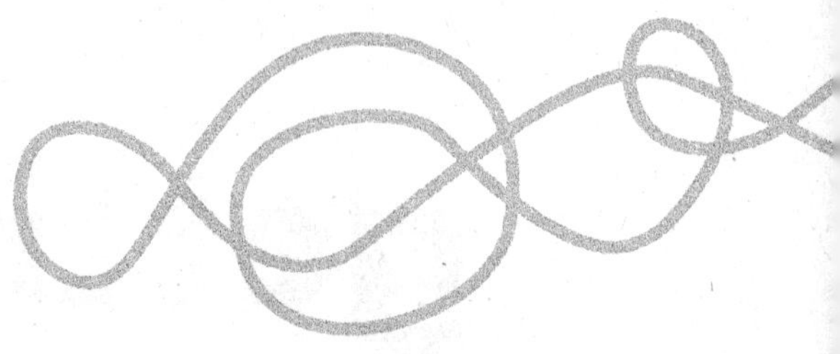

Congratulations on taking this journey. You've already taken a courageous first step. In Part One of this workbook, you will discover more about your Self and your parts.

There are many ways to tell your Self from your parts. In this section you will get to practice some common ways to distinguish the two. Parts can, and often do, carry burdens and hurt from the past. Self cannot be damaged. Self continuously radiates Calm, Clarity, Confidence, Curiosity, Connectedness, Creativity, Compassion, and Courage (the 8 Cs). Parts fluctuate and can display helpful and harmful behaviors. Self is you at your core. Parts are exactly that, just a part of you. You can recognize when you're "in a part" because it's usually playing a role to protect you. When you're not exhibiting those attributes related to your Self—the 8 Cs—a part is generally present.

You will have an opportunity to learn to speak for your parts and use IFS to get to know your parts. These practices will lay the groundwork for you as you begin this healing journey.

Trust your Self-energy. Stay open and curious. Enjoy the journey!

an invitation to go within

We spend so much time in the external world, looking at screens, seeking outside validation. What would happen if we spent more time inside ourselves? This practice is an invitation to go within. This is the first step to assessing your parts. To get to know your Self and parts, you will need to become familiar with going inside yourself. You can follow the guide here to practice going inside.

- Find an inviting space or a comfy chair.
- Close your eyes to remove any distractions.
- Take a few deep breaths.
- Notice what comes up inside you. Are there certain thoughts, emotions, sensations, or parts that show up? Are there nervous parts? Impatient parts? Agitated or indifferent parts? Skeptical or hopeless parts? Let them know they are all welcome.

- Focus on each part one by one to see which parts may be present in your internal system.
- Move to curiosity. Stay open to any part or feeling that shows up.
- When you're ready, come back to the outer world and open your eyes.

Take five minutes to try these prompts for going inside. When you're done, answer these questions.

Did it feel comfortable or uncomfortable for you to go inside?

What thoughts, feelings, or sensations came up, if any? If nothing came up for you, that's okay too. This is just the beginning. Follow the guides and prompts in the rest of the workbook and trust the process.

discovering your self

Before now, you may not have realized that there is a difference between your Self and your parts. Remember, your Self cannot be damaged. Your Self has the compassion needed to heal the parts in your inner system. Parts can overwhelm you and run the show until they learn to trust your Self. In this exercise, you will explore the differences between the attributes of your Self and the parts that are in your inner system.

Take some time to reflect on attributes of your Self that have been a constant throughout your life.

These are the qualities you would associate with your truest, most authentic Self. This could be some of what we call the 8 Cs:

Calm, Clarity, Confidence, Curiosity, Connectedness, Creativity, Compassion, and Courage

or other attributes like honesty, trustworthiness, playfulness, or kindness. See what feels authentic to you.

In the circle below, list as many attributes of your Self as you can:

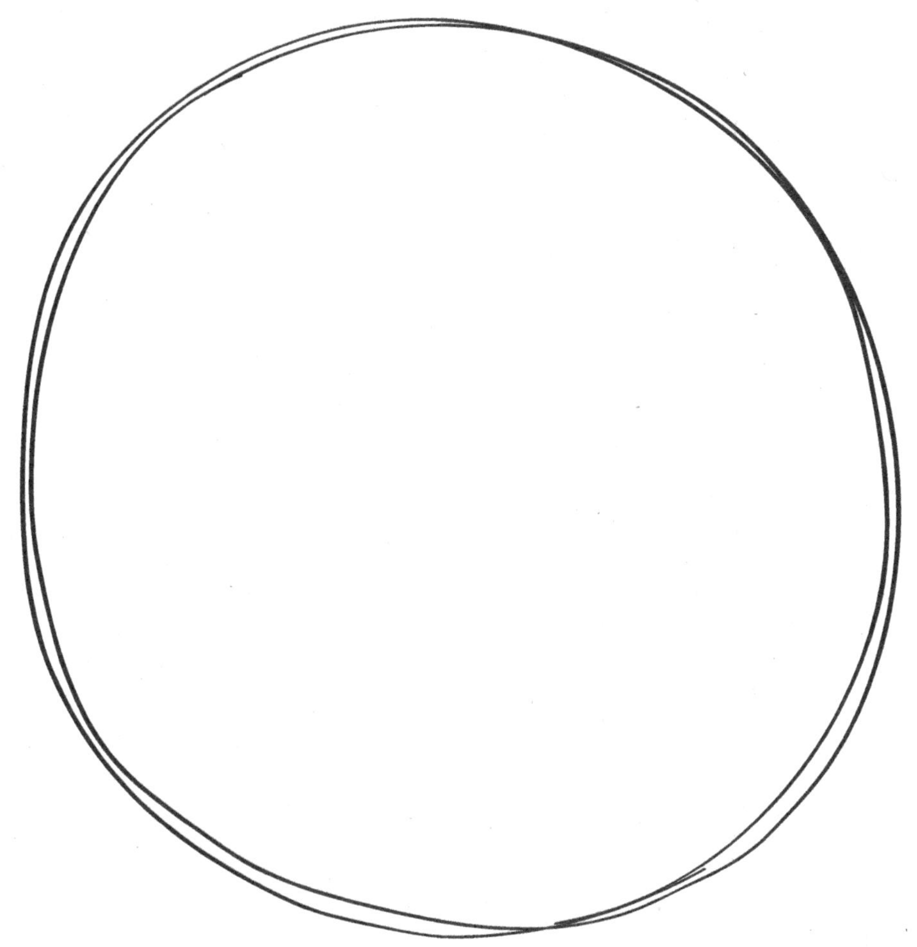

Reflect on a few moments in your life when you were exhibiting one or more of the 8 Cs of Self (Calm, Clarity, Confidence, Curiosity, Connectedness, Creativity, Compassion, and Courage) and write them in the boxes:

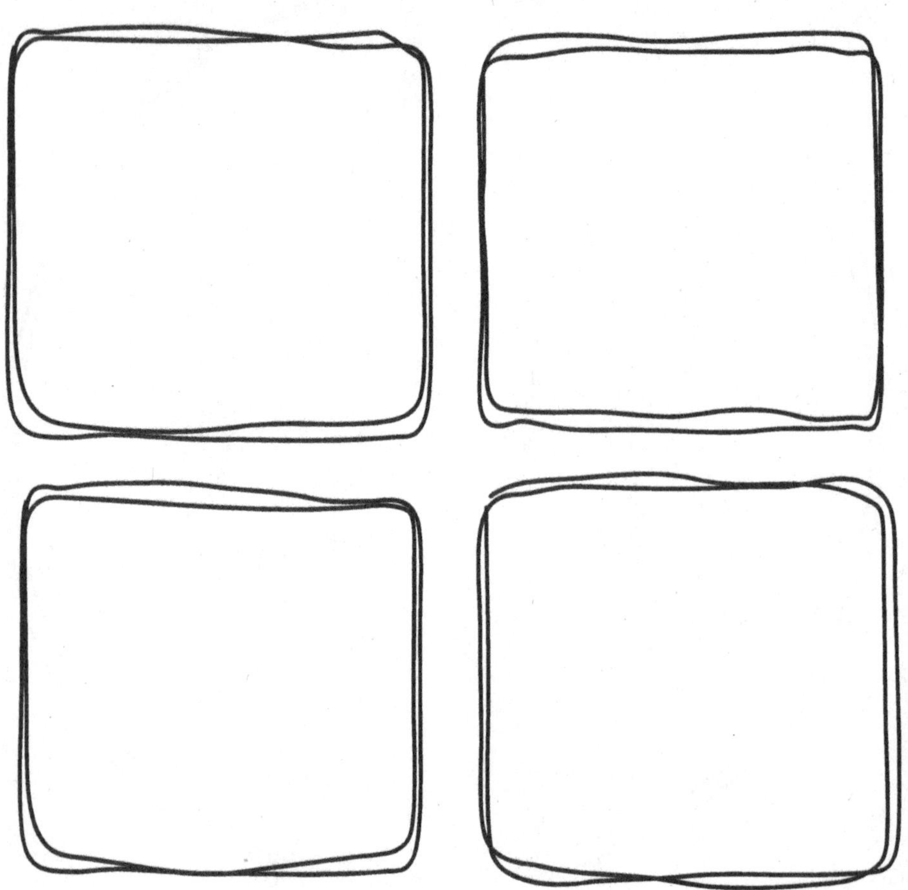

What did it feel like in those moments to be connected to your Self? Did you feel peace? Love? Hope? Energy?

What do you feel now as you reflect on those moments?

the difference between self and parts

Now that you are familiar with the qualities of Self, it will be easier to tell the difference between when Self is leading and when parts are taking over. Remember, you can recognize when you're "in a part" because it's usually playing a role to protect you. When you're not exhibiting those attributes related to your Self, a part is generally present.

→ **Reflect on some attributes or behaviors that you've noticed in yourself that aren't characteristic of your Self and write them in the boxes.**

These might be impatience, irritation, jealousy, laziness, distractedness, depression, worry, etc.

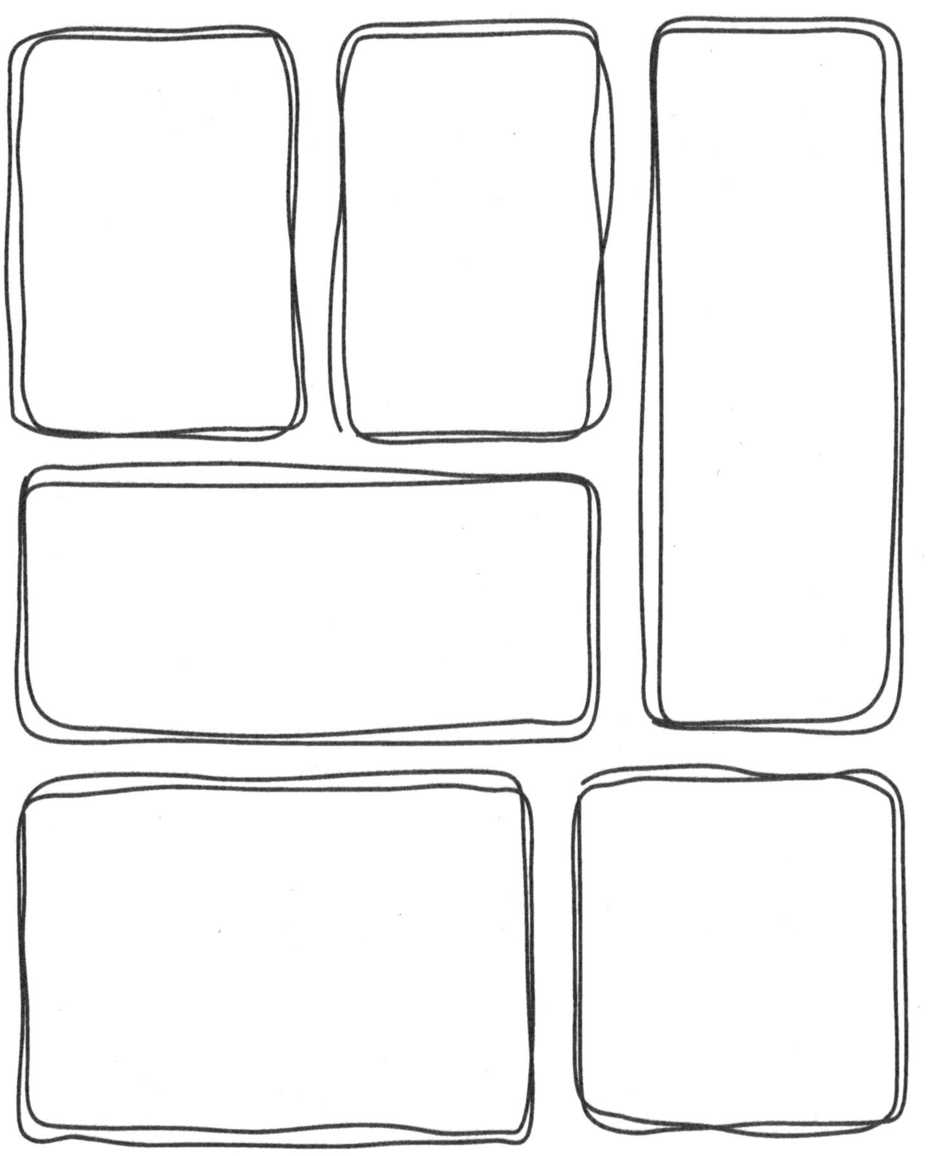

Reflect on some significant moments when these parts have shown up in the recent past. Write down a few moments you can recall on the lines below.

When you were acting out of these parts, how did you feel toward these parts?

How did others react to these parts?

one part: a meditation

Meditations can help you access your Self and grow curious toward your parts. This meditation is designed to help you get to know a part that you want to help or change your relationship with. Maybe you feel anxiety in your chest before you speak in front of a group, or you wish you didn't feel shy when meeting someone new—these are examples of trailheads that lead us to our well-meaning parts An audio recording of this practice is available at:

soundstrue.com/the-ifs-workbook-bonus

Take three deep breaths.

Think of a part that you would like to get to know better or help understand. This could be an anxious or worrying part, or maybe a perfectionistic or people-pleasing part.

Select one and focus on it.

See if you can find it in or around your body.

If you can't, that's okay.

Focus on however you experience this part, whether it's a sensation, feeling, or thought.

As you focus on it, notice how you feel toward it.

If you feel anything toward it besides at least curiosity or acceptance, then find the parts that are giving you other feelings (anything other than the qualities of Self). See if they're willing to relax for a little while and not interfere, so you can just get to know the one you started with.

Assure these other parts that you won't let the part take over, you're just going to get to know it a little bit.

See if you feel a little curious about this original part.

You may find that the other parts won't step back. That's okay. You can spend time getting to know their fears about stepping back from the original one instead.

But if the parts do let you get curious about the original one, then it's safe to get to know it in the way that feels right to you.

It may just want to know why you want to know about it. It may want to communicate what it's been trying to do for you or what it might need from you.

Allow some time to get to know this part. See what questions it has for you.

After a few minutes, thank the part for letting you know what it did. Let it know this doesn't have to be the only chance. They can always come back to you another time.

Before you come back, be sure to thank the other parts for letting you get to know this one or letting you know they were afraid to.

When that feels complete, take a couple deep breaths again and come back to the room.

getting in touch with your emotions

Are you in touch with your emotions or is it a challenge to identify what you're feeling? Getting to know your parts can help you get more in touch with your emotions and vice versa. There may be a part or parts blocking you from feeling your emotions. You may have parts that feel annoyed or angry at you for even going through this workbook. That's okay. Emotions are messages from our parts, and in order to understand them, we first need to notice them. When you start this work, there will probably be a lot of parts trying to get your attention. That's totally fine. In the same way that you can have a wide range of emotions, you can also have many parts.

In this exercise, you'll have the opportunity to explore the emotions within your internal system.

Take some time to read the emotions on the wheel and answer the questions that follow.

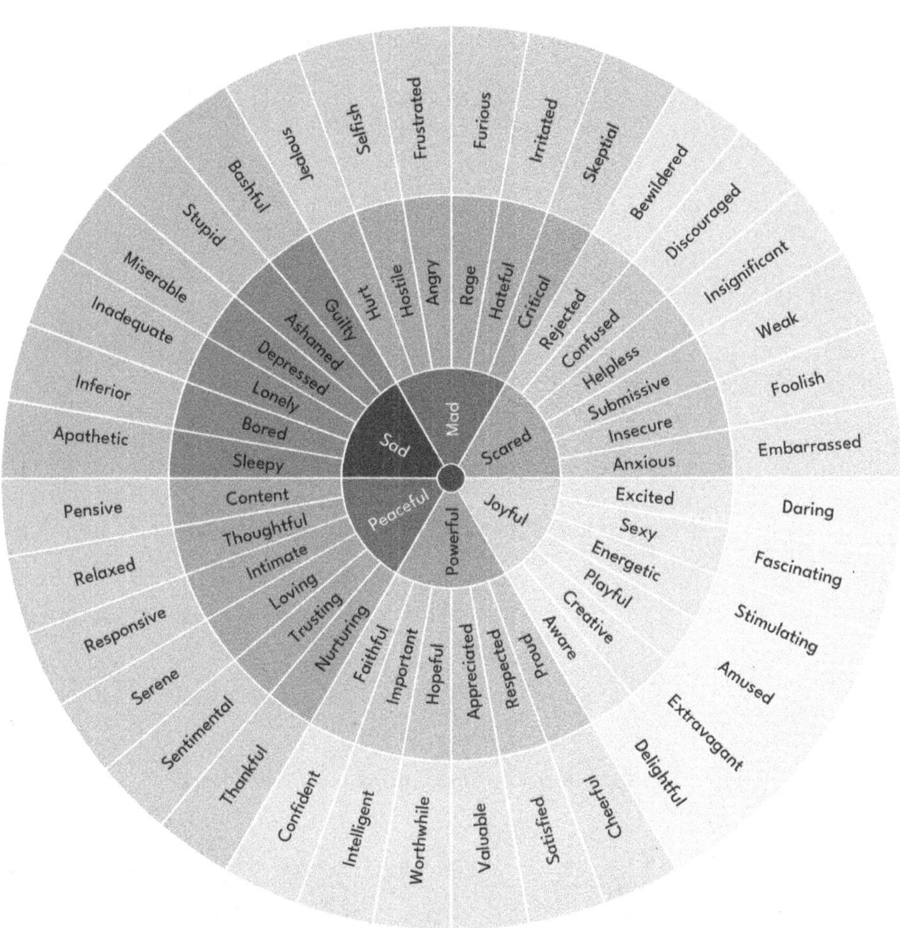
Sad
Mad
Scared
Joyful
Powerful
Peaceful
Guilty
Ashamed
Depressed
Lonely
Bored
Sleepy
Hurt
Hostile
Angry
Rage
Hateful
Critical
Rejected
Confused
Helpless
Submissive
Insecure
Anxious
Excited
Sexy
Energetic
Playful
Creative
Aware
Proud
Respected
Appreciated
Hopeful
Important
Faithful
Nurturing
Trusting
Loving
Intimate
Thoughtful
Content
Bashful
Stupid
Miserable
Inadequate
Inferior
Apathetic
Jealous
Selfish
Frustrated
Furious
Irritated
Skeptial
Bewildered
Discouraged
Insignificant
Weak
Foolish
Embarrassed
Daring
Fascinating
Stimulating
Amused
Extravagant
Delightful
Cheerful
Satisfied
Valuable
Worthwhile
Intelligent
Confident
Thankful
Sentimental
Serene
Responsive
Relaxed
Pensive

What emotions from the wheel have you felt in the last . . .

Day	Week	Month

What section of the wheel do you feel the most?

What section of the wheel do you feel the least?

What specific emotions from the wheel do you rarely, if ever, feel?

What emotions would you like to feel more?

Take a moment to go inside. What emotion(s) are you feeling right now?

find, focus, and flesh out

This exercise helps you connect with your parts using six steps called the 6 Fs: Find, Focus, Flesh Out, Feel Toward, BeFriend, and Fear. You will practice the first three in this exercise and the other three in the exercises to follow. You may recall some of these steps from the previous meditations. Take your time going through these steps. Oftentimes, parts will emerge spontaneously as you turn your attention inward.

These steps may feel unusual at first. Don't worry. Use emotions and internal feelings and sensations as your clues. They will guide you to your target part(s). You will have the opportunity to practice using these steps throughout the workbook. You may need to return to this exercise whenever you want to connect with a part. Eventually, these steps will become second nature, much like a spiritual practice.

Follow the steps to connect with one of your parts. Write down anything you learn in the blanks.

Find

- Go inside and see if any thoughts, emotions, or sensations come to your attention.
- Take these sensations as coming directly from the part that wants your attention in this moment. This will be your target part.

Write down any thoughts, emotions, or sensations from the part that came to your attention:

Focus

- Focus on the part that you just found by giving it your attention.
- Spend time with the part and let the part reveal itself to you in whatever way it chooses.

Write down anything that the part shows you:

Flesh Out

Now flesh out the part by asking your Self these questions:

- Where does this part show up in or around the body?
- What sensations or emotions do you feel, if any? Are there any images that come up?

Don't judge the process if not much came up this time. Once you feel comfortable with the steps, you can try this exercise again and again. Next time, see if you can do the steps with your eyes closed. Don't worry about writing anything down. Just really try to be present to any parts that show themselves.

feel toward

After you identify your target part, it's time to see how you feel toward the part. The purpose of parts work is to bring your parts into relationship with your Self so they can be healed. This step is a crucial one because it lets you know if you are accessing Self or have other parts that are getting in the way. If you're feeling anything other than the 8 Cs (Calm, Clarity, Confidence, Curiosity, Connectedness, Creativity, Compassion, and Courage), that is a good indicator that another part is present. You can ask parts to step back so you can get to know the target part. If they relax and step back, thank them. If they don't, ask them why not. If your parts are not able to step back, you can return to this exercise when they may feel more ready. Don't push your parts. They will let you know when they're ready. These exercises help parts build trust in your Self. Just as in other relationships, trust takes time.

For the purpose of this exercise, identify your target part. It could be the same part as the last exercise or a new one that reveals itself. After you've focused and fleshed it out, follow the prompts below and write your answers in the space provided.

Feel Toward

How are you feeling toward this part as you get to know it?

Is your heart open or closed to this part?

Check for Self-energy

- If you notice the presence of the 8 Cs (Calm, Clarity, Confidence, Curiosity, Connectedness, Creativity, Compassion, and Courage) you can continue with the last two steps.
- If you feel anything other than the 8 Cs, it's likely another part showing up. Ask this part if it can step back while you connect with the target part.
- If it steps back, thank it and go back to the "Feel Toward" step above. If it doesn't step back, ask it why not. Come back to this exercise when your parts feel ready.

Write anything you've learned here:

One way to build trust with parts is to reassure them that you want to get to know them. When you ask a part to step back, you can let them know you will connect with them later. When you finish the steps with the target part, you can go through the steps again with any other part that comes up. Be careful not to overpromise anything to your parts. If you tell them you'll check in later, make sure to follow through. This will help you build their trust.

befriending and fear

To help your parts, you need to be in relationship with them. When you know your Self-energy is present, you can go on to befriending your part. In this exercise, you'll be locating a new part and letting it know how you feel so they can relax and open up to you. (For example, you might say in your mind or out loud, "I feel tenderness for you," or "I feel curiosity about you.") When they feel your compassion, they will tell you whatever you need to know about them. This will give you valuable insight so you can understand and relate with your parts. An overworking part may feel like they are neglected or unappreciated. They might tell you what age they started overworking or let you in on the good intentions behind their actions.

Using the steps from the previous two exercises, find a new target part and focus, flesh out, and feel toward the part. If your Self-energy is present, you're ready to follow the next step. Write your answers in the spaces.

BeFriend

- Extend compassion, kindness, and comforting words to the part to create a connection between your Self and parts.
- Notice how the part responds.
- As the part feels comfortable with you, it will begin to tell you about itself.
- What role does this part play for you? How are they trying to protect or help you?
- Does it like its role?

What did your part(s) tell you?:

Fear

- Sometimes parts are afraid to stop their roles, or they don't trust you. Ask your part what would happen if they stopped, or why they don't trust.
- Thank the part for being open with you. Make a plan to check back in with the part at a later date.

Write down anything you learned:

the path: a meditation

This meditation will help you differentiate your Self from your parts by using a path as a metaphor to locate parts of yourself. Accessing Self is a continual process required by parts work and essential for healing your parts, but it takes practice. This meditation is yet another invitation to meet Self. An audio recording of this practice is available at:

soundstrue.com/the-ifs-workbook-bonus

Take a deep breath.

In your mind, put yourself at the base of a path.

It could be a path you've been on before
or one that is completely new.

Just stay there at the base for a minute.

Before you go anywhere, meet with your parts and
let them know you are going to walk by yourself.

If they have any fears, you can let them know you won't
be gone long, but this will be good for them and you.

You can ask the ones who aren't afraid
to comfort the ones who are.

Still, you may find that there are parts
that don't want you to go.

Spend some time listening to their fears.

If they don't want you to go, respect their wishes, and come
back to this meditation later when they do feel ready.

If they are okay waiting for you, then head out
on the path, at whatever pace feels right.

As you go, you'll be asked to notice a few things. The first
thing: Are you *on* the path or *watching yourself* on the path?

If you're watching yourself, there's a
part that's trying to do it for you.

Ask that part to be willing to return to the base
and let you continue being on the path.

As you go along, also notice if you're thinking anything.

If you're thinking anything at all, it usually means there's a part still with you.

Find those parts and see if they'd also be willing to wait at the base.

If they are willing, you'll gradually notice you're having a purer experience of awareness.

As you go, if you find at any point, you are flying or soaring, that's okay, it's fine. Just go with it.

Notice your body. You might find a vibrating energy running through it.

See if it's possible to hold that energy. This is Self-energy.

As you feel that vibrating energy, you can pause and see if it has anything to say to you.

When the time feels right, return to the base. There is no rush.

When you get back to your parts, meet with them to see how that felt for them. See if they'll let you hold this energy while you're away.

When that feels complete, thank them for letting you go, if they did. Or you can thank them for letting you know they were afraid.

Take two or three deep breaths and come back to your chair.

a part of me feels . . .

When using the IFS model, it is helpful to use "parts language" to communicate what's going on inside your system. Instead of stuffing emotions or letting emotions take over your inner system, you can speak for the part that is feeling the emotion the most intensely. You can say, "A part of me feels angry at what you just said," or "I have a part that is sad you weren't there for me." This may seem unusual at first, but speaking about our parts in such a way trains us to distinguish our Self from our various parts every day as a practice. In this exercise, you'll learn to use "parts language" to communicate the emotions your parts are feeling and what is going on inside you.

Read the situations and complete the statement using parts language.

Example: The house is a mess and you are feeling like a failure.

A part of me feels *like a failure because the house is a mess.*

Situation 1: You have deadlines approaching and you are feeling waves of anxiety.

A part of me feels ______________________________

Situation 2: You have an internal conflict because you feel like someone is taking advantage of you.

A part of me feels ______________________________

Situation 3: You're being asked to work overtime again and you're exhausted.

A part of me feels ______________________________

Name three situations in the last week when you had a strong reaction to something and write a response using parts language.

Situation 1: ______________________________

A part of me feels ______________________________

Situation 2: ______________________________

A part of me feels ______________________________

Situation 3: ______________________________

A part of me feels ______________________________

speaking for, not speaking from: part 1

When emotions arise, they are felt across your whole inner system of parts. The emotion may be coming from a part or parts, and by speaking for that part, you are able to realize it is only a part and not the totality of who you are. This gives you some space to understand what is happening and better communicate with others your wants, needs, and fears. You are able to speak *for* your parts, not *from* them.

When you speak *for* your parts, you are able to speak with confidence and offer clarity. Speaking *from* parts without awareness of what is happening inside can cause confusion, conflict, and harm. In this exercise, you will learn the difference between speaking for parts and speaking from parts.

See if you can tell the difference between speaking *from* a part and speaking *for* a part. Read the examples, then label whether the statements are speaking "from" or "for" parts.

Examples:

Speaking from: You're always on your phone!

Speaking for: I have a part that really wants to connect with you.

Speaking from: What's the point in talking, nobody cares what I have to say.

Speaking for: I have a part that wants to know you care.

1. *Speaking* __________: How could you be so thoughtless and lose track of time? Now we're going to be late.

   Speaking __________: I have a part that's disappointed you lost track of time. I really wanted to get there early.

2. *Speaking* __________: I have parts that feel overwhelmed by all that needs to get done, could you please help?

   Speaking __________: Do I have to do everything around here?

3. *Speaking* __________: Part of me is frustrated and needs some space. Can we talk later?

   Speaking __________: Don't talk to me, I can't deal with you right now.

4. *Speaking* __________: I am about to lose it.

   Speaking __________: A part of me feels overwhelmed. I need some space to process my emotions.

Answer Key: 1. from, for; 2. for, from; 3. for, from; 4. from, for.

speaking for, not speaking from: part 2

Now that you are able to distinguish between speaking from parts and speaking for parts, let's go deeper. In this exercise, you will have the chance to apply what you've learned to your own life. You can use this language anytime to describe charged situations and emotions, and see how, over time, it helps to create space between Self and your parts.

Think of a situation where you had a strong reaction.

What would you say in the moment *from* a part?

Now, what would you say in the moment if you were to speak *for* the part?

Going Inside Take a moment to bring some awareness to the emotion, bring some compassion to the emotion. If your part is still highly charged after speaking for the part, that's okay. This isn't easy. Use the skills you've learned. Go inside. Find, Focus, and Flesh Out the part. Befriend and bring some kindness to the part. In time, the emotion may shift.

real-world scenarios

Using parts language is an essential foundation, and learning to speak for your parts is the key to distinguishing between your Self and your parts. In this exercise, you will put into practice what you've learned about speaking for parts in a variety of real-world scenarios.

In the following real-world scenarios, come up with at least two alternative responses.

Example: Someone keeps talking over you in a conversation.

I have a part that is frustrated that I keep getting interrupted.

A part of me feels disrespected because you keep talking over me.

Your friend forgot to call you on your birthday.

You have been diagnosed with an unknown illness and you are feeling apprehensive.

A family member is acting passive-aggressive and using biting sarcasm.

You're having a disagreement about money with a loved one and you want to check out.

You want to go home but your friends want to stay out.

You are not sure how you feel but you notice your system is being activated.

Someone mispronounces your name again.

You are told how brave you are, but you are actually feeling terrified.

Your child brought home a report card with a failing grade.

mapping your parts

It's time to explore further and identify some of the other parts that are in your internal system. At first, you may have a hard time distinguishing parts because this is a new way of thinking about yourself. The more you practice IFS, the more you'll be able to identify different parts. Knowing your parts gives you greater Self-awareness and allows you to heal parts that may be carrying hurts and burdens. Before you can heal parts, you need to identify them.

Take some time to reflect on the parts that you've been able to identify and connect with so far in the workbook.

Think about parts that may have surfaced in the assessment, meditations, or exercises. You can include other parts that you were aware of before you started this workbook. Remember, all these parts are welcome.

Examples of parts: a part that distracts you when you have a deadline; excited or apprehensive parts; an overachieving or perfectionistic part; or young parts that have been caretaking for family members or grieving from a loss. You can describe the parts however you want. Sometimes parts will let you know what they prefer to be called. Take time to listen to each part.

Map your parts by writing them down or drawing them in the space below:

IFS Tip

Parts mapping can be enhanced by using creative tools. If it feels right, gather some colored pens or markers, play some music you like, sit outside under a tree or cut out some pictures from magazines. These tools may help your parts express themselves more fully.

a one-minute daily check-in

Here's a really quick check-in you can do anytime or anywhere to start to learn about your system. Consider trying this for one or two minutes a day. It's a simple practice that can have a positive impact on how you feel. Your parts will feel more comfortable showing themselves, knowing you are interested and wanting to connect with them. This quick check-in can help you feel more connected to your parts throughout the day and for your parts to build trust with you.

Stop.

Notice what's there. Perhaps it's an emotion or disturbance.

See if you can open yourself to it.

Let the parts know you're there to connect with them.

Ask your parts what they want to tell you. Don't think—just wait for the answer.

Thank your parts for anything they share with you.

This is a mini-meditation you can do any time to access your inner system and locate the parts of you that need attention, so you can tend to them as a regular practice. Remember, you don't have to be perfect, just be present.

part two

appreciating your overworked managers

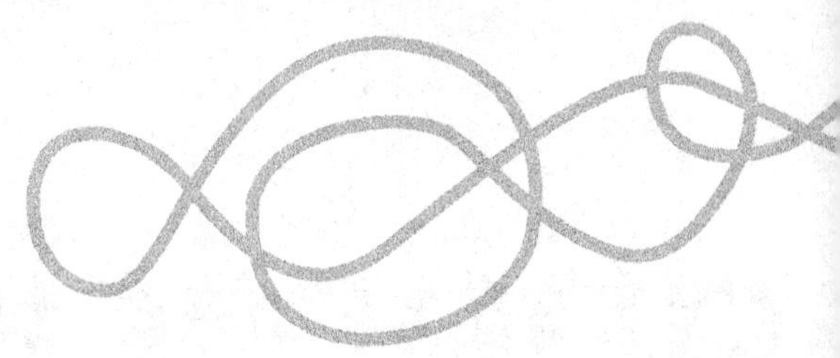

You have done some important work so far. You have laid a foundation to really build on. You have learned to go inside, connect with Self, and BeFriend your parts. You've learned to speak for parts using parts language. This is foundational work for the journey ahead.

In Part Two, you will meet your manager parts. Managers are protector parts that desperately want to keep you out of trouble. They do this in a number of both helpful and harmful ways. Manager parts act preemptively to shield you from emotions, pain, and/or shame. These parts order and control your life so you can be liked, loved, and respected.

Manager parts, like all parts, bring helpful qualities to your life, too. They help you stay up all night to cram for an exam. They make to-do lists so you can get things done and be productive. When managers run the show, however, they can keep you anxious and stressed, and work you to the point of burnout. It's important to remember that protector parts mean well but their intention often isn't apparent. Frequently, you notice them because of the impact they have on you and others. Once you understand their intentions and fears, you are able to befriend managers and partner with them in balanced and healthy ways.

Don't forget to check back inside to see how your internal system is doing periodically as you go through the workbook.

You may have overachieving or perfectionistic parts that really want to hurry through the exercises to feel affirmed. Remind those parts that it's not just about the destination, it's the journey.

your internal managers self-assessment

This is an assessment of behaviors commonly associated with manager parts.

On a scale of 1 to 5 (1 = rarely, 5 = commonly), rate how often the behaviors show up in your life.

___ I make to-do lists to feel accomplished and organized.

___ I get a lot of worth from what I do.

___ I feel out of control if I don't have a plan.

___ I live by the mantra "practice makes perfect."

___ I often work after hours.

___ I feel uncomfortable when other people don't have a plan.

___ I feel like everything depends on me.

___ I'm the glue that holds my family together.

___ I remember birthdays and other significant dates.

___ My house is spotless.

___ I schedule vacations months in advance.

___ I push myself and others hard.

___ I'm never satisfied with my performance.

___ My mind is always thinking about what else can be accomplished.

___ I try to anticipate worst-case scenarios.

___ I like using spreadsheets to track my activities.

___ I try new diets and fitness programs to achieve better results.

___ I say yes even when I want to say no.

___ I look for apps that help me take control of my life.

___ I judge others who are late or disorganized.

___ I have trouble trusting others to do things I ask them.

___ I get stressed out when I'm working on projects because I want to do it right.

___ I pay attention to deadlines and strive hard to meet them.

Total # of 5s: ___

Total # of 4s: ___

Total # of 3s: ___

Total # of 2s: ___

Total # of 1s: ___

If your 5s and 4s are highest, you have very active manager parts.

If you have a lot of 3s, you have somewhat active manager parts.

If your 2s and 1s are highest, you have manager parts, but they may not be as active.

all parts welcome: a meditation

In IFS, all parts are welcome. There are no bad parts. Parts are well intentioned even when they take on extreme roles that end up doing more harm than good. The behavior may have bad consequences, but the parts are not bad. Parts are often very young, parentified parts doing the best they can to protect and care for you. Once you understand that these parts mean well and often work tirelessly to support you, you are able to show them compassion and connect with them through your own Self-energy. For this exercise, you are invited to follow the meditation to welcome all your parts. An audio recording of this practice is available at:

soundstrue.com/the-ifs-workbook-bonus

To begin, get in a comfortable seated position.

If you would like to close your eyes, you can.

Take a couple of deep breaths.

Try to locate your Self in your body.

Bring the qualities of your Self to mind and see if you can feel your Self-energy.

When you sense a strong connection to your Self, take some time to remember the different emotions and parts you've been reflecting on throughout this workbook.

Tell those emotions and parts they are all welcome.

Perhaps you want to put your hand on your heart.

You may say internally or out loud, "All my parts are welcome."

Repeat it a few times.

Notice how your parts respond.

When you're ready, open your eyes.

who's the boss: exploring manager parts

Our parts are trying to protect us but due to trauma we may have experienced, they often feel they need to take over and run the show with the best of intentions. Proactive protectors or managers are vigilant parts who try to prevent your inner exiles (vulnerable parts) from being activated and your internal system from being flooded with emotion. They're hardworking parts that employ various strategies (from demanding to criticizing or even shaming) to keep you on task and out of your body and emotions.

It's important to keep in mind, this isn't the essence of the part. These are just the roles those parts have been forced into, like a kid who finds themselves in a parentified role or over their head because of the dynamics of the family. While the child might be very critical of their siblings, it's not the essence of the child to be that way. It's the role they were forced into for perceived survival. In the same way, parts are like parentified children simply trying to do their best to protect you.

Strategies commonly associated with manager parts are:

Circle the parts that you have noticed inside you. Add any additional strategies of your manager parts in the space below.

Perfectionism	Worrying	Overworking
Criticizing (inner critics)	People-pleasing	Intellectualizing
Restricting food	Overexercising	Caretaking
Controlling (of you or others)	Hypervigilance	Fastidiousness
Frugality	Building up walls	Bossiness
Busyness	Legalism	Performing
Codependency	Stuffing emotions	Micromanaging
Overly judgmental	Overfunctioning	Competitiveness
Blending in	Playing small	Over-accommodating
Overachieving	Extreme planning	Overanalyzing
Overcommitting	Catastrophizing	Phobias
Dissociating	Repressing sexuality	Avoiding conflict

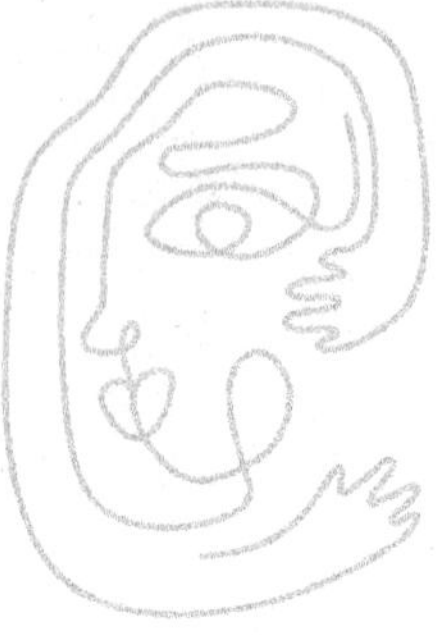

Going Inside Take a pause and go inside to see if any parts are reacting to this exercise. Are there parts feeling frustrated, judged, or shamed? Close your eyes. See what parts show up. Find a part and focus on it. Let them know they aren't alone and that you are there to listen to them. If you are feeling overwhelmed by a part, see if the part will step back so you can continue. Reassure them that they are welcome in your system and that you desire to connect with them. If they step back, thank them.

IFS Tip

When asking a part a question, try not to think about what it might say. Just listen for the part to respond. This takes practice! Many of us have strong thinking parts who want to step in or explain.

it's the thought that counts

Parts are well intentioned. They really are trying to protect you and the most vulnerable parts of you. Manager parts are hard workers. When healthy, they can help you achieve incredible things without taking over your life. When you're able to understand and appreciate the ways they are trying to help you, you are able to feel more compassion for them and show them the appreciation they are longing for. When they feel your presence and love, they will be able to trust you more and not need to drive the bus. When they have more opportunities to meet the Self, they will over time feel more comfortable quieting down and trusting the Self to lead more of the time.

For this next exercise, you're going to identify the good intentions behind your parts.

You can do this by going inside and asking the part directly how it's trying to help you, or ask it what it's afraid would happen if it didn't do what it does inside you. In answering that question, you will often learn how it's trying to protect you.

Part	**Good Intention**
Example: *A perfectionistic part that hates to mess up.*	*This part wants me to be successful, respected. This part thinks that by pushing me to become the best, I can be loved and avoid feeling like a failure.*

strengthening relationship: a meditation

Here's a meditation to strengthen your relationship with one of your parts. Since our parts don't really know us, sometimes it takes a little while for them to feel comfortable telling us about themselves. This meditation offers an opportunity to find a part to be in a relationship with and get to know it. You'll start to feel what the part feels like in your body, and then develop a relationship with it by letting it know that you're genuinely curious. An audio recording of this practice is available at:

soundstrue.com/the-ifs-workbook-bonus

Close your eyes.

We're not trying to do anything, we're just trying to notice what's there.

Maybe you notice a thought or a sensation.

You may notice a whole bunch of thoughts, sensations, or parts, and that's okay.

If you notice more than one, just see which one is calling to you the loudest.

Maybe you're curious to get to know what one of these things is. Just pick one.

Once you find the part, focus on it, and see if you can tell how you feel toward it.

If there's anything other than the 8 Cs present (the Self), see if the other parts will step back.

Get curious about who this is.

If it feels okay, let them know you're curious.

Let curiosity radiate toward them. Invite them to feel that curiosity. See how they react to that.

Now we're befriending.

Stay with this; it's about making this part comfortable.

They're starting to get to know you.

When they're comfortable being with you, then they'll let you know about them.

They can tell you their story.

They can tell you anything they need you to know about who they are, including what they are afraid would happen if they didn't do what they're doing.

befriending a manager

Like the meditation in the previous exercise shows us, there is more than one way to befriend and get to know a part. It takes practice and this exercise is another entry point.

Take some time to get to know one of your manager parts using the steps you learned (on pages 36–44).

Choose a manager part you identified in a previous exercise that you are curious to get to know.

- Find, focus, and flesh out a manager part you'd like to befriend.
- How do you feel toward the part?

Check for Self-energy:

Do you notice the presence of the 8 Cs (Calm, Clarity, Confidence, Curiosity, Connectedness, Creativity, Compassion, and Courage) or similar feelings? If yes, you are ready to befriend.

If no, there's a part interfering. Ask that part if it's willing to relax or step back while you work on the target part. If it is, return to the "feel toward" question. If it is not willing to step back, ask it why not. You can return to this exercise when your parts feel ready.

- Spend time befriending the part.
- Create a Self-to-part connection by extending compassion, kindness, and comforting words to the part.
- Notice how the part responds.

Write it down here: ______________________________

- As the part feels comfortable with you, it will begin to tell you about itself.

Write down anything it wants to tell you:

What else does the part want or need from you?

What role does this part play for you?

Find out what the part is afraid would happen if it didn't do this role.

Thank the part for being open with you. Make a plan to check back in with the part at a later date. Use this exercise anytime you detect the presence of a manager part.

interviewing a part

Now we're going to take our curiosity and relationship-building a step further. Learning to interview your parts is an essential way to discover more, not only about the part, but yourself. Try to stay non-judgmental toward the part. Be curious about what they might want to share with you. You might be surprised by what you learn.

Select one of the parts from the previous exercise or another part that shows up. Then answer the questions related to this part.

If you notice other parts jumping in, ask those parts if they're willing to step back and give you some space. After you complete this exercise with the target part, you can run through it again with other parts.

Example:

- The part I would like to get to know is *a caretaking part.*
- Describe this part in a sentence: *This part feels responsible for the happiness of all my family and friends.*
- Where does this part show up in the body? *My shoulders.*
- When did this part start doing this role? *When I was young, maybe eight years old.*
- What are the drawbacks of this part? *I neglect myself because I'm so focused on everybody else.*
- What are the benefits of this part? *This part helps me show care and love to others.*
- What role does this part play for you? *It helps me feel useful to people and keeps me busy so I don't have to deal with my own pain and issues.*
- What do you appreciate about this part? *I appreciate that it wants to protect me from my own pain.*
- How do you feel toward this part now? *I feel compassion.*

Now it's your turn:

The part I would like to get to know is

Describe this part in a sentence:

Where does this part show up in the body?

What are the drawbacks of this part?

What are the benefits of this part?

What role does this part play for you?

What do you appreciate about this part?

How do you feel toward this part now?

You can run through this same exercise with one or two other parts:

The part I would like to get to know is

Describe this part in a sentence:

Where does this part show up in the body?

What are the drawbacks of this part?

What are the benefits of this part?

What role does this part play for you?

What do you appreciate about this part?

How do you feel toward this part now?

what are you afraid of?

Manager parts are often driven by fear. Fear can drive managers to overfunction, causing burnout and other detrimental side effects. In this exercise you will look at fears commonly associated with manager parts.

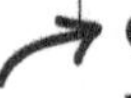

Check the fears that your manager parts resonate with:

- ❍ Being overwhelmed by emotions
- ❍ Becoming like your parent(s)
- ❍ Looking stupid
- ❍ Being rejected
- ❍ Feeling judged or shamed
- ❍ Falling short
- ❍ Disappointing people or yourself

- ❍ Not being good enough
- ❍ Embarrassing yourself
- ❍ Chaos and disorder
- ❍ "Negative" or scary emotions
- ❍ Feeling out of control
- ❍ General catastrophe
- ❍ Feeling pain or shame

Are there other fears your manager parts may have?

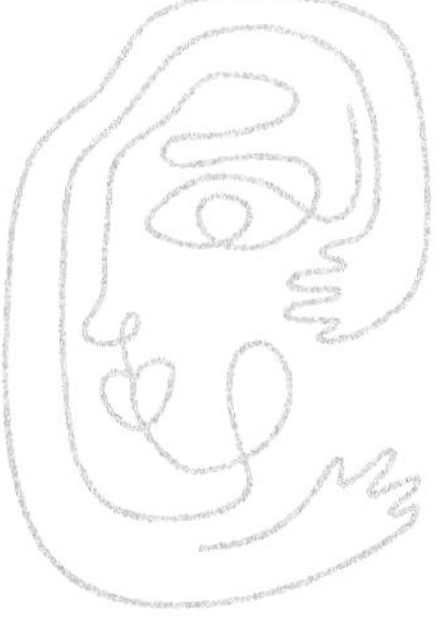

Going Inside One important question to ask your manager parts is: "What are you afraid would happen if you stopped doing this role?" What is an inner critic part afraid would happen if it didn't point out your flaws? This will let you know what is important to it and why it works so hard to push you. Take a moment to connect with one of your manager parts. Ask it what it's afraid of. See what it says.

showing a little appreciation for managers

Manager parts work hard for you. They help you meet deadlines, they keep you organized, and they keep you motivated. Even when they overfunction or take on extreme roles, they really do mean well. One way to build a relationship with them is to acknowledge their good intentions and show them appreciation. Showing a little appreciation can go a long way to build trust and connection. When parts feel affirmation from Self, they are less likely to look externally for validation. Managers, like all parts, need connection to your Self to be healed.

In this exercise, you will have an opportunity to show your appreciation for your hardworking manager parts.

What are one or two manager parts you'd like to show appreciation to?

What do you appreciate most about these manager parts?

How have they protected you?

How have they come through for you in clutch moments?

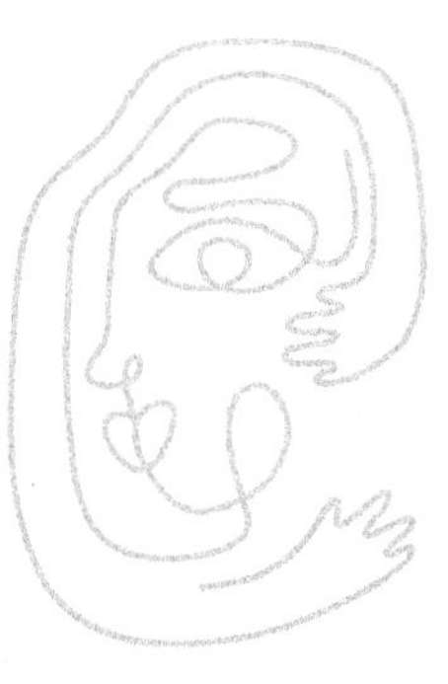

Going Inside Take a moment right now and share the appreciation you feel toward your manager parts. If you are feeling positive feelings toward this part, then extend some love and compassion. You can speak the words out loud or inside yourself. You might say, "I really appreciate . . ." or "Thank you for the ways you have . . ." If you're not feeling positive feelings, that's okay. You can try again another time when you do feel sincere positive feelings.

embodiment: a meditation

IFS is an embodied practice, which means it incorporates your whole body. It's common for parts to manifest in different areas of the body. For example, an anxious part might manifest in the chest. Paying attention to the body is a way to get in touch with parts. In this meditation, you are going to locate where a part is in your body. An audio recording of this practice is available at:

soundstrue.com/the-ifs-workbook-bonus

Take some deep breaths.

See what parts are present.

Scan your body for places of tension, achiness, congestion, stiffness, or pressure. Often those are what we call *trailheads* (manifestations of parts that are present).

You can also scan your mind for agitated thoughts or emotions. Look for any inventory of who is there right now.

As you notice a trailhead or part, focus on it in that place in your body or mind.

The goal of this meditation isn't to get to know it, but to let it know it's not alone.

As you focus on it, let it know you're there with it.

If it's possible, in a sincere way, let it know that you care about it. Even if it's a part that gets in your way in life.

You can do that by giving it some comforting words or extending a loving energy to it or around it.

You could even breathe into it.

Do one or all of those things until the part seems to relax.

If it does relax, you'll notice a shift in your body or mind in the direction of more space.

If it doesn't relax, that's okay, it just needs more attention from you at another time.

For now, you can let it know you understand, and you'll return to it when you have more time, and you can move on to a different part.

If it does relax and you feel that increase in spaciousness, then move on to another part, extend loving energy to it or a comforting word, helping each of these parts know they are not alone.

You are with them, and they can trust you. They can trust you to be in your body.

As they relax and you enjoy more spaciousness, you might notice a kind of energy flowing in that space, in and around your body.

You can shift your attention between the energy as it flows back and forth from your Self to the part, bringing more of that Self-energy to them.

Notice the vibratory quality of the energy or the sense of well-being that comes with it. The sense of faith and calm.

You can now begin to shift your focus back to the outside world. See if it's possible to hold this spaciousness and awareness even as you begin that shift.

With practice, it's possible to be in this state even when you focus outside and interact with other people. Eventually, your parts will grow to trust you to lead them in this way.

When the time feels right, come back to the outside world.

find it in the body: managers

Building off the previous meditation, this exercise will help you practice finding a part in your body. It can be difficult to find a part in the body and it takes practice. At first, it can feel quite abstract and removed, but it gets easier. Noticing what's happening in your body is important so that you don't get stuck in your head. Remember, IFS is an embodied practice. Finding the part in your body will help you connect with your body and your parts.

Choose a manager part that you have felt this week (critical, perfectionistic, worrying, caretaking, overworking, people-pleasing, etc.) and map where you feel them in your body on the picture.

Go inside to find the part. Notice if you feel the part anywhere in the body, including your head. And, if you can't, don't worry. It takes practice. Try again later.

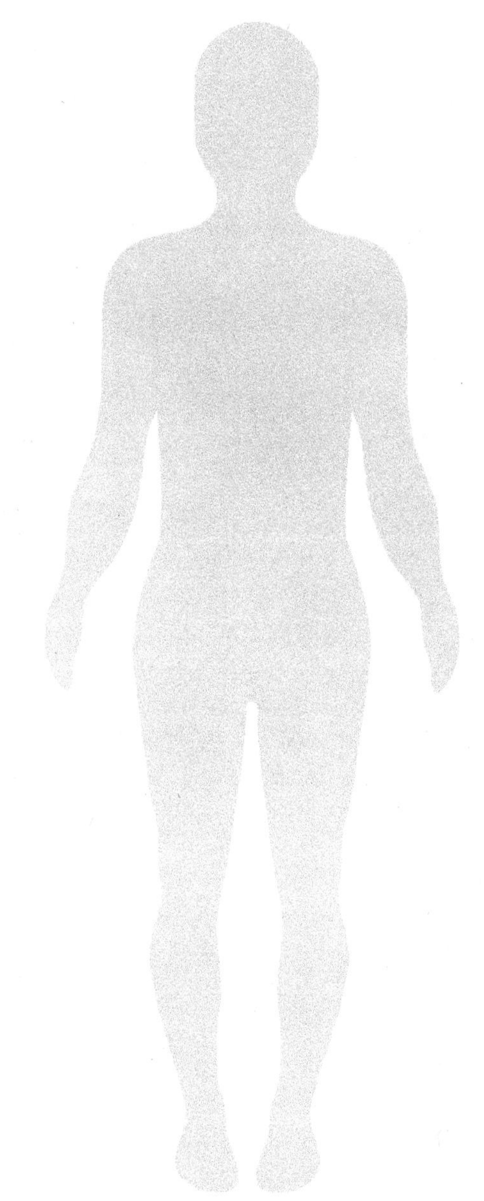

checking in with an inner critic: a meditation

The inner critic parts, like all your parts, are trying to help you. As a child, you may have been bullied by other children, hurt by a loved one, or shamed by authority figures. The inner critic is often formed through a childhood trauma. An experience doesn't have to be life-threatening or dramatic to be experienced as a trauma by a part. A part's trauma might come from living with an abusive parent, but it could also come from an embarrassing moment, a critical teacher, or feeling left out of a group. These formative experiences may not seem so traumatic on the surface, but when you were a child, you experienced significant pain from them; these young parts are still hard at work trying to protect you from feeling that old pain or trauma. The inner critic parts think their role is to point out flaws to avoid trauma, embarrassment, ridicule, or punishment. They think they must continue playing this role even when you're older, because they are frozen in the time when it happened and believe you are still young. This meditation invites you to befriend your inner critics and appreciate how they are trying to help. An audio recording of this practice is available at:

soundstrue.com/the-ifs-workbook-bonus

Close your eyes.

Try to locate an inner critic part in or around your body. Maybe it's a tightness in your chest or a literal pain in your neck.

Get curious about this part.

What thoughts, feelings, impulses, or images are connected to this part?

Stay open to what this part may want to show you.

As this part brings a feeling or image to your mind, see how you feel toward this part.

If you have enough curiosity, let the part know you want to hear more.

Be open for what the inner critic may want you to know about it.

Ask the part how old it thinks you are.

If it thinks you're younger than you are, update the part on your age now.

Ask the part how old it is.

Ask the part what role they've been playing for you.

Let the part know you appreciate how they have been trying to help you.

If you are feeling any compassion, love, or tenderness toward this part, let it know.

See if the part has anything else it wants to tell you.

If not, you can return to the space.

Open your eyes.

part three

befriending your activated firefighters

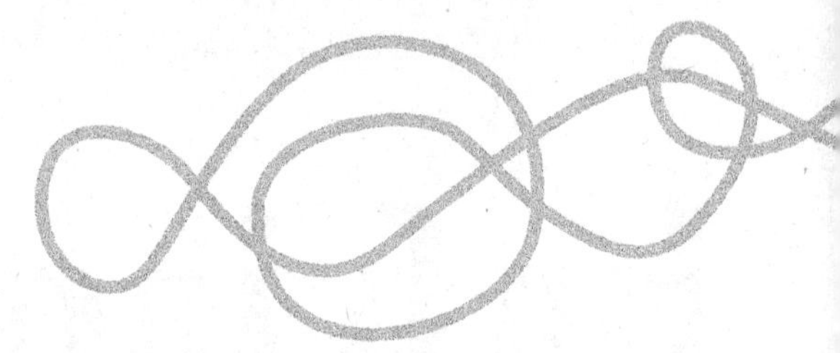

In the previous section, you connected with some of your manager parts, listened to them, and befriended them. You are on a path of healing. Way to go! Simply taking a few minutes to go inside and connect with your parts can make a huge difference. Hopefully, you and your parts have already noticed a positive change. If you haven't, that's okay, too. Keep going! Stay open and curious.

In this section, you are invited to explore your firefighter parts. Like managers, they are protective parts. Whereas managers work preemptively to avoid and control emotions, firefighters react when your deep pain is triggered. Firefighter parts step in to protect you when you are activated or experiencing trauma. Their job is to rush in and rescue you (and your vulnerable parts) from pain by any means necessary. Their goal is to put out the fires of uncomfortable emotions. They may do this in a number of ways such as soothing, confronting, fighting, numbing, or dissociating.

Firefighter parts are related to habits or impulses. You can change habits and impulses by changing your relationships with these parts. Befriend your firefighter parts, listen for their good intentions, and show them you love them even when they act out.

Understanding and showing compassion to firefighter parts is another essential step in your healing journey.

your internal firefighters assessment

Mark an "X" next to any of the following behaviors that you have engaged in the last twelve months.

- ❍ Had an emotional outburst that you regretted.
- ❍ Cursed in your head or out loud when you felt pain.
- ❍ Binge-watched an entire season of a show over a weekend.
- ❍ Consumed alcohol to forget about your problems.
- ❍ Lost your temper with a family member or pet.
- ❍ Did some retail therapy.
- ❍ Engaged in sexual activity as an escape from harder emotions.
- ❍ Had a heated argument with someone.

- ❍ Used food to numb your feelings.
- ❍ Felt road rage.
- ❍ Fantasized about getting revenge.
- ❍ Engaged in destructive behavior.
- ❍ Dissociated during the day.
- ❍ Escaped into imagination or fantasy to avoid reality.
- ❍ Smoked a pack of cigarettes in a day.
- ❍ Slept in past noon.
- ❍ Frequently went to the movies.
- ❍ Tuned out by watching sports.
- ❍ Ate lots of sweets to make yourself feel better.
- ❍ Made big impulsive spending decisions.
- ❍ Scrolled through house or job sites looking to make a big change.
- ❍ Acted out of character.
- ❍ Left a person or business a 1-star review because you were treated poorly.
- ❍ Got irritated with a customer service representative.
- ❍ Screamed into a pillow.
- ❍ Went off on someone you love about something unrelated.
- ❍ Did something incredibly adventurous or risky.

- ❍ Scrolled for hours on social media.
- ❍ Went on an extravagant vacation.
- ❍ Had a mental, emotional, or physical affair.
- ❍ Chewed out a coworker.
- ❍ Thought about quitting your job.
- ❍ Made a high-risk bet or financial gamble.
- ❍ Slammed a door or abruptly walked away during a heated conflict.
- ❍ Gave someone the silent treatment because they hurt you.
- ❍ Argued with someone on social media.

Total # of Checks: ____

If you have 0–5, your firefighter parts are rarely active.
If you have 6–10, your firefighter parts are sometimes active.
If you have 11–15, your firefighter parts are often active.
If you have 16–20, your firefighter parts are very frequently active.
If you have 20+, your firefighter parts are extremely active.

firefighters to the rescue

Reactive protectors, aka firefighters, want to help you escape an emotionally overwhelming situation. They want to keep your vulnerable exiles protected at all costs. They will go to extreme lengths to pull you out of a situation. While the managers seek control in order to keep you safe, firefighters seek to numb, soothe, and distract in order to ease the pain. Firefighters want to bring immediate comfort, relief, pleasure, and/or escape from painful emotions.

Read through the list of strategies commonly associated with firefighters. *Circle* the firefighter strategies that your parts have engaged in.

Confronting (fight)	Leaving (flight)	Drinking to soothe
Vegging out on TV	Playing video games	Eating sweets
Explosive outbursts	Lashing out	Feeling strong
Dissociating	Risk taking	Extreme sports
Escaping into fantasy	Gambling	Procrastinating
Addiction	Egotism	Promiscuous behavior
Overindulging	Excessive spending	Driving recklessly
Attention-seeking	Flirting	Acting violently
Overmedicating	Binging shows	Skipping class or work
Cutting off relationships	Oversleeping	Scrolling social media
Bullying	Excessive traveling	Pursuing toxic relationships
Chasing the high	Seeking gratification	Checking out
"Retail therapy"	Affairs	Avenging
Shutting down	Self-harming	"Us versus Them" mentality

Add any other firefighter strategies you've noticed inside your system.

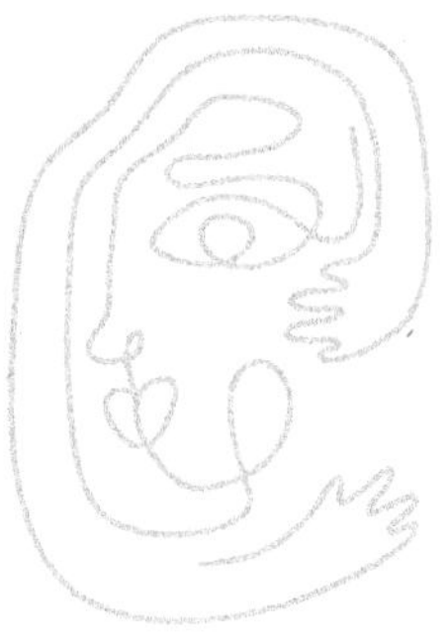

Going Inside Take a pause and go inside to see if any parts are reacting to this exercise. Are there firefighter parts reacting to these behaviors? Or are there manager parts that fear or hate them? Can you get those managers to relax so you can get curious about the firefighters? Do they want you to know anything else about them? Close your eyes. Let them know you are there to listen to them. If you are feeling overwhelmed by a part, see if the part will give you some space so you can continue with this workbook. Reassure them that they are welcome in your system and that you desire to connect with them.

IFS Tip

Some firefighters have extreme behaviors, including self-harm. If your firefighters use extreme behavior to take you away from your emotions, and they become activated with these exercises, they may need support from a friend or mental health professional. You can also skip any part of this workbook that feels too overwhelming.

all parts welcome, all behaviors are not

It's sometimes hard to separate the part from the behavior. While all parts are welcome, all behaviors are not. Using the IFS model helps us see the difference between a part's intentions and the extreme behaviors or outcomes it produces. The goal isn't to get rid of these parts, but to understand and embrace their intentions with compassion.

In this exercise, you're going to practice separating the good intention from the problematic behaviors.

↗ **Using the firefighter parts you have identified already, fill in their good intentions and problematic behaviors.**

Part	Good Intention	Problematic Behavior
Example: *A fighting part*	*protects you from harm*	*hurts people, pushes them away*

find it in the body: firefighters

It's common for firefighter parts to manifest in different parts of the body. A firefighter part might manifest as physical cravings or impulses. A firefighter part may seek comfort in food when activated. Paying attention to the body is a way to get in touch with parts. In this exercise, you are going to locate where a part is in your body.

Where do you feel firefighter parts in your body?

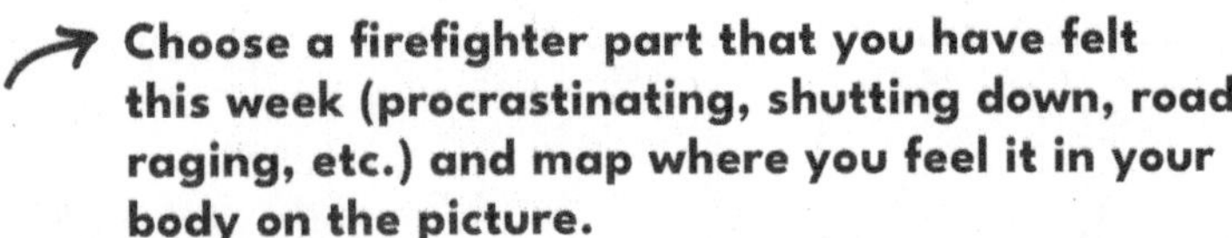

Choose a firefighter part that you have felt this week (procrastinating, shutting down, road raging, etc.) and map where you feel it in your body on the picture.

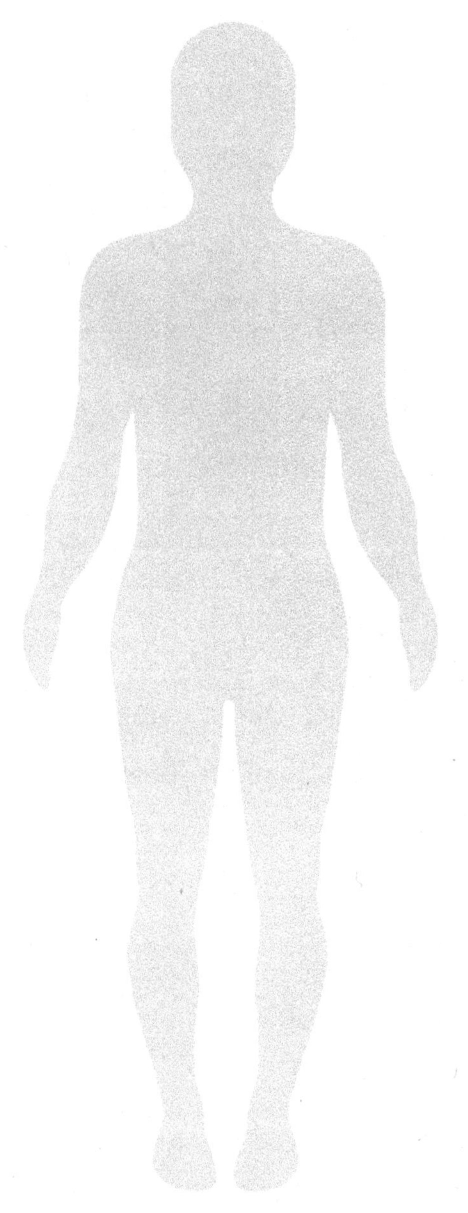

firefighter meditation

Healing happens when parts connect with your Self and feel the qualities of Self. In this meditation, you will spend time connecting with one of your firefighter parts. Pay attention to what sensations you feel in your body and how this part responds to you. An audio recording of this practice is available at:

soundstrue.com/the-ifs-workbook-bonus

Get in a comfortable position. Take three to five deep breaths to slow down and go inside.

Notice what is supporting your body and where your body is touching the ground.

When you feel ready, select a firefighter that you have some curiosity about.

Try to clear your head of any preconceived ideas about them.

Notice where they may be present in your body.

How close are they to you?
Do they want to get closer?

Are there any other parts that are feeling apprehensive about you connecting with your firefighters?

Can you ask them if they are willing to step back for a moment? Let them know you are curious to get to know them too, another time.

When you've identified the firefighter part, see if there's a word, image, sensation, or impulse they want to show you.

Try to stay curious.

How are you feeling toward this part?

If you feel compassion, extend it to this part. If you don't feel compassion or curiosity, that's okay. You may need to ask a judgmental or criticizing part to step back.

Remember your parts are like children. They are scared and in over their heads.

They are doing the best they can to protect you.

See what you're feeling toward them now. If you're feeling compassion or connectedness, let the part know.

Let them know you appreciate their efforts to rescue you. Tell them you want to connect with them. They are not alone.

See if there's anything else they want you to know about them.

If they tell you anything, thank them. If they didn't tell you anything, that's okay. Thank them for just being with you.

When you're ready to return to the room, you can open your eyes.

befriending a firefighter

Remember, befriending is a foundational skill of IFS. Just like you practiced with other parts, now you have an opportunity to befriend a firefighter part on your own.

Recall a recent situation when one of your firefighters was activated.

- Find, focus, and flesh out a firefighter part you'd like to befriend.
- Notice where it shows up in or around your body.
- Notice any thoughts, feelings, sensations, or images.
- How do you feel toward the part?

Check for Self-energy:

- Do you notice the qualities of Self or similar feelings? If yes, you are ready to befriend.
- If no, it's likely a part interfering. Ask the part if it's willing to relax or step back while you work on the target part.
- If the part is willing to step back, return to the "feel toward" question. If it is not willing to step back, ask it why not. You can return to this exercise when your parts feel ready.

Befriend

- Spend time befriending the firefighter part.
- Create a Self-to-part connection by extending compassion, kindness, and comforting words to the part.

Notice how the part responds. Write it down here:

As the part feels comfortable with you, it will begin to tell you about itself. Write down anything it wants to tell you:

What else does the part want or need from you?

What role does this part play for you?

Find out what the part is afraid would happen if it didn't do this role.

Thank the part for being open with you. Make a plan to check back in with the part at a later date.

what are they protecting?

Firefighters are protectors. They take on their protective roles when you're young to keep you safe. In this exercise, you will explore what your firefighter parts are protecting you from.

Use the firefighter parts you've already identified to answer what each part is protecting you from. Use the IFS practices you've been learning to go inside and connect with each part.

If another part steps in while you're working with the target part, you can ask the part to step back momentarily. In other words, be sure you're experiencing some of the 8 Cs as you get to know the protector.

Firefighter Parts	What are they protecting you from?
Example: *Overeating*	*Sad feelings, remembering past wounds*

coming in hot

Firefighters can disrupt our lives and relationships. These extreme actions are well intentioned but damaging nonetheless. They signal to us that healing is still needed. Often, they are trying to capture our attention or remove us in the quickest way possible from a triggering or traumatic situation. What can you do when your firefighters are activated? The IFS model helps you speak for these parts, so you can help yourself and others know where the feeling or behavior is coming from. You can take time to understand the firefighters to learn when they started functioning in these roles and what they are afraid would happen if they stopped.

In this exercise, you are going to learn four steps to take when you want to de-escalate a firefighter when they are coming in hot.

Step 1: Slow Down

Step 2: Get Curious

Step 3: Speak for Parts

Step 4: Use These Moments as Trailheads for Future Exploration

What are ways to slow down when you're feeling activated? Ex. count to ten, take three to five deep breaths, ask the part to separate from and trust you to handle the situation, get curious.

What are ways to get curious? Ex. ask the part why it's so upset.

How can you speak from Self for your part? Ex. I have a part that is really angry you misunderstood me and I'm learning that it protects a younger part that was often misunderstood.

What future trailheads does this situation provide? Ex. I want to take some time to explore my explosive-anger part in my next counseling session.

the fun parts

Firefighters can get a bad rap for getting us into trouble, but they're not bad. Believe it or not, when released from their extreme roles, they are the fun parts. They keep your life exciting, providing much-needed balance to your overachieving and hardworking manager parts. Without firefighters, your life would be boring, and you'd never rest. You'd also be less likely to set boundaries or stand up for yourself. Firefighter energy can be helpful in situations when you need a firm "no," the room needs a good laugh, or you need to infuse some play into a stale daily routine. In this exercise, you're going to have some fun with your firefighters.

List the good, clean fun your firefighters provide in the following areas.

Examples might include adding spontaneity, needed snack breaks, or enjoyable activities to look forward to after work; reminding you to play and pursue creative outlets; adding spice and excitement by trying new things, etc.

Everyday life:

Work:

Family:

Spirituality:

Intimate relationships:

Friendships:

Community:

Vacations:

Hobbies:

Finances:

Charity work:

showing a little appreciation for firefighters

Firefighter parts can cause friction in relationships and with authority figures or institutions. They are the parts that might embarrass you when they act out or show off. They frustrate your managers, who work hard to keep them under control. This may leave your firefighter parts feeling shamed and unloved, which will only cause them to act out more.

In this exercise, you will have an opportunity to show your appreciation for these parts.

Firefighters, like all parts, need connection to your Self to be healed.

What are one or two firefighter parts you'd like to show appreciation to?

How have they brought more joy and fulfillment to your life?

How have they protected you?

What positive results have you experienced from risks they've made you take?

Going Inside Take a moment right now and share the appreciation you feel toward your firefighter parts. If you are feeling positive feelings toward this part, then extend some love and compassion. You can speak the words out loud or inside yourself. You might say, "I really appreciate . . ." or "Thank you for the ways you have . . ." If you're not feeling positive feelings, that's okay. You can try again another time when you do feel sincere positive feelings.

fire drill: a meditation

Are you ready to connect with one of your firefighters? In this meditation, you will have the opportunity to get to know some of your firefighter parts and show them appreciation for how they've been protecting you. An audio recording of this practice is available at:

soundstrue.com/the-ifs-workbook-bonus

Take a few deep breaths.

Think of a person in your life who really seems to activate you—a person who triggers all kinds of protectiveness inside you.

This could be a family member, someone you work with, or even a celebrity of some kind.

In your mind's eye, put that person in a room by themselves. You're in another room watching them from a window.

As you watch that person, have them do the thing that activates you and notice the parts of you outside the room wanting to protect you or reacting in a vulnerable way to this person.

You may only notice one in a big way or there may be a whole room full of them out there with you.

You don't have to go into the room with the person at all. You're just going to spend some time getting to know these parts. See if you can get curious about them.

Let's start with the ones that want to protect you.

Spend a little time with this part and ask: What are you afraid would happen if you show up with this person, if you didn't try to step in front of me or have to deal with this person?

See if in that conversation, you can show them appreciation for how hard they work to protect you from people like that. How hard they have worked to keep you safe.

You can also learn about the parts that protect you from this person.

That may be enough to learn about these protective parts. You can spend some more time continuing that. But if it feels safe, you can take it one step further and ask if the protective parts would be willing to let you enter the room, while they stay outside. The parts could watch through the window if they wanted. See if they are willing to let you go in and be with this person—not so the person will change, but just to see how it goes and let you handle them as an experience. Again, there's no pressure to allow that if it doesn't feel right.

But if they give permission, go ahead into the room and notice how you are feeling without this part. Interact with the person in whatever way feels natural.

As you are interacting, if you sense one of your protective parts coming in, see if it's possible for it to trust you and go outside. Reassure that part that you can handle it.

Whenever the time feels right, you can go back to your parts outside the room and see how they react. See how they think you did. You might also want to know how willing they are to let you do this in the outside world with this person.

When all that feels complete, you can begin to shift your focus back to the outside world and open your eyes.

on guard: responding to other people's firefighters

Once you are able to show compassion for your parts, you will better be able to show compassion for other people's parts, especially when they resemble your own. This can help you resolve conflicts more peacefully and can also help deepen your relationships with other people. Understanding how your firefighters respond to trauma and uncomfortable emotions can keep your heart open and keep you curious toward others. In this exercise, you will learn how to stay curious when other people's firefighters are activated so that you can remain calm in a conflict.

Look at the following scenarios and write down ways you can respond to other people's firefighter energy.

Scenario 1

Your friend lost a close family member.

You offer to talk with them about it and they snap at you for bringing it up.

What might be going on for them?

The grief is painful, and their firefighter is lashing out because it's afraid of feeling the sadness of the loss.

What might be going on for you?

You feel hurt that your efforts to console were not welcomed.

How can you respond with compassion?

I understand this is a lot for you to process. I have parts that want you to know I'm here if you need support. We can talk about it later when you're ready.

Scenario 2

A family member is drinking excessively the night before a big job interview. You are worried they will drink too much and not do well in the interview, so you try to get them to stop drinking. This makes them agitated and storm off.

What might be going on for them?

What might be going on for you?

How can you respond with compassion?

Scenario 3

Your boss is stressed and goes off on you and your coworkers for not meeting a deadline.

What might be going on for them?

What might be going on for you?

How can you respond with compassion?

Scenario 4

Your child lashes out at you because you limited their phone time.

What might be going on for them?

What might be going on for you?

How can you respond with compassion?

part four

embracing your burdened exiles

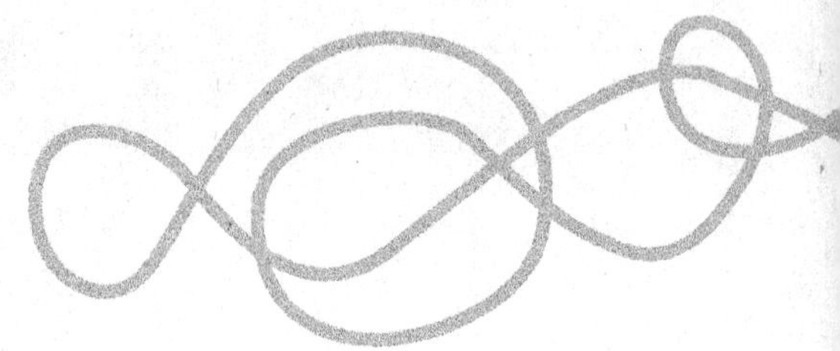

You are doing really important internal work. Give yourself a pat on the back for your bravery and commitment to make it this far. You have connected with your manager and firefighter parts. You've gone inside, connected to parts, and put the IFS skills into practice.

In Part Four, you will have the chance to get in touch with your most vulnerable younger parts: exiles. We all have exiled parts or what some might call *inner children*. Before they're hurt, they are open, playful, and innocent. Because they are sensitive, they get hurt the most by the things that happen to us. When they get hurt, terrified, or feel ashamed and carry these burdens, some of our parts don't want anything to do with them because they make us feel bad all the time. We tend to lock them away.

When you have a lot of exiles, you feel more delicate, the world feels more dangerous, and other parts have to shift out of their natural qualities to become protectors. Many of them are parentified children. Like in a family, the older siblings often take on parental roles, but they aren't equipped even though some of them seem very wise and confident. There's not one exiled child, but many, and they are stuck in different scenes and carry different burdens. Connecting with your inner exiles can be the most life-changing experience. These are young, hurting parts in need of love and healing.

In this part, you will have the opportunity to extend love to these tender parts.

Remember, go at your own pace. Only do what feels safe enough for your system. Be sure to check in with your system regularly. If you notice protector parts jumping in, return to some of the previous exercises until they feel ready.

exiles inventory

In this section, you will explore some of the emotions and fears your exiled parts feel.

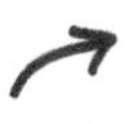

Read through the list of inner messages and then go inside to see what your exiles fear is true about them. *Circle* the one(s) that your inner exiles feel the most strongly.

I am bad.

I am unlovable.

I am unworthy.

I am worthless.

I am overwhelming to others.

I am helpless.

I am hopeless.

I am powerless.

I am painfully sad.

I am terrified.

I am guilty.

I am stupid.

I am a failure.

I am lost.

I am all alone.

I am my worst mistake.

I am unwelcome.

I am unwanted.

I am rejected.

I am an annoyance.

I am an embarrassment.

I am a mistake.

I am a problem child.

I am a mess.

I am damaged.

I am broken beyond repair.

I am deficient.

I am damned.

I am cursed.

I am evil.

I am garbage.

I am nobody.

I am not seen.

I am not valued.

I am misunderstood.

I am not important.

Are there any other emotions or fears your exile parts may feel that are not listed above?

How do you feel toward your exile parts knowing they feel this way?

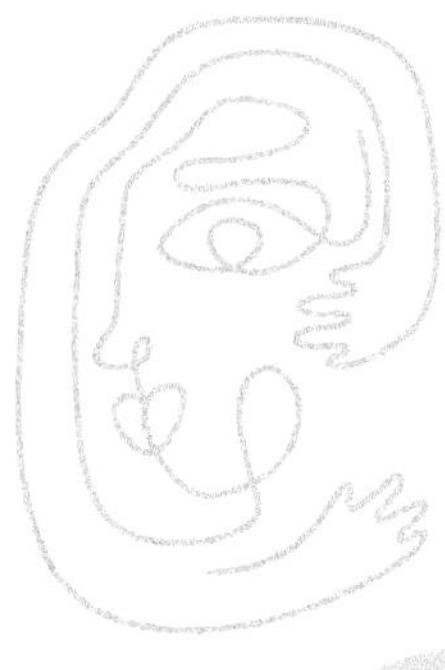

Going Inside Take some time to attend to your parts. If you are feeling Self-compassion and -energy, speak comforting words to your exiles.

IFS Tip

Healing using IFS can take many forms. While healing exiles is the deepest work, it can take time (in some cases, years), working with your protective systems—and possibly with the support of a mental health professional—before your system will allow access to exiles. This is very normal. It is not a failure—your system is working to protect you. Much healing can take place by working to deeply listen to and understand your protective system.

heart: a meditation

This might be a good time to check in on your heart. In this meditation, you will explore how open or closed your heart is. This might be challenging for your parts. Don't push to make anything happen. If it feels like too much you can stop at any point. An audio recording of this practice is available at:

soundstrue.com/the-ifs-workbook-bonus

Start by taking a couple deep breaths.

With this meditation, we'll start by having you focus on your heart, however you experience it.

This doesn't have to be your exact physical heart, but however you experience your heart.

As you focus on it, get to know it in a physical way.

We're going to explore different qualities of your heart to see what kind of condition it's in.

The first thing I invite you to notice is how open it is versus how closed.

Check to see how tender it is versus crusted or calloused.

How congested is it, versus fluid and flowing?

It's also interesting to notice how much space it has in there.

Does it feel really contracted and tightly packed, or spacious?

You might find in your exploration that different places in your heart are different in quality.

Maybe the front is closed and the back is open, or the top is tender and the bottom is tough.

Maybe energy can flow through part of it but not other parts, or maybe in some places it feels tense or contracted, and in other spaces it's spacious.

Where it feels closed, contracted, or calloused, it means there are some protective parts manifesting.

If you'd like, you can take a second to get to know those protectors.

You can get a little curious about what they're afraid of.

Open your heart fully to allow it to be tender.

Did the protector parts try to contract? Answering that question, they'll teach you about vulnerable parts in your heart or around your heart.

Right now, you don't have to go to those parts, but just get to know them from the protectors.

Also, it's possible to get to know how vigilantly they've been protecting your vulnerability.

Extend a loving energy for how hard they've worked, or needed to work, to protect your heart.

See how they react to that appreciation.

Right now, we're not asking them to change anything about that or expecting them to.

We are just getting to know their fears and showing them appreciation.

You could propose that, at some point in the future, they could let you go to those vulnerable parts so you could heal them. Then the protectors could relax and allow you to open your heart.

Often, they don't believe that healing is possible. They feel they must guard your heart in this way for your protection.

You can just let them know that it is possible but there's no pressure to do it.

When this work with the protectors of your heart is through, you can shift back. Before you leave, be sure to thank them for letting you know this, and how hard they have worked to keep your heart safe.

find it in the body: exiles

It's common for exile parts to manifest in different places in the body, or even outside it. An exiled part might manifest as a pit in your stomach, as an impulse of dread, or in your heart as tightness or fear. Paying attention to the body is a way to get in touch with parts. Where do you feel exile parts in your body?

→ **Choose an exile part that you have felt this week ("I am worthless," "I am sad," "I am so scared," etc.) and map where you feel them in your body on the picture.**

If nothing comes to mind, that's okay. You can return to this exercise at any time.

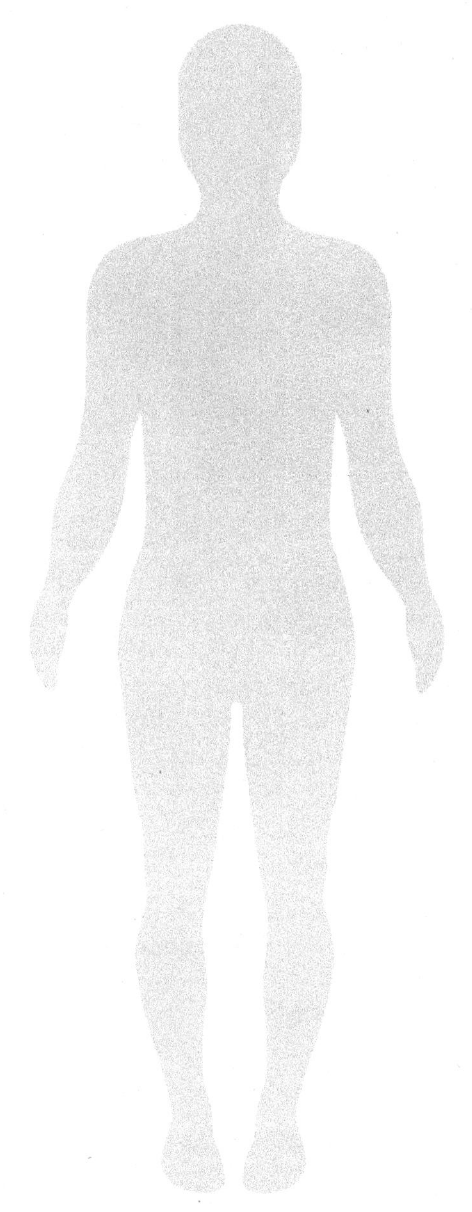

the story of your life

One way to identify exile parts is to look back on your life story. By revisiting significant memories and moments in your life, you can notice patterns and parts that you may have not seen before. In this exercise, you are invited to reflect on the significant moments that defined you as a way to witness your own story. Notice what happens in your inner system as you reflect on different moments. You might feel sadness or a sensation in your body as you move from one scene to another. Be aware of any emotions or messages that may be connected to the events.

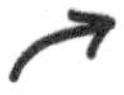

Draw your life story. In each box, draw a significant life event or memory.

Ex. a milestone birthday, a graduation, a big move, the death of someone close, etc.

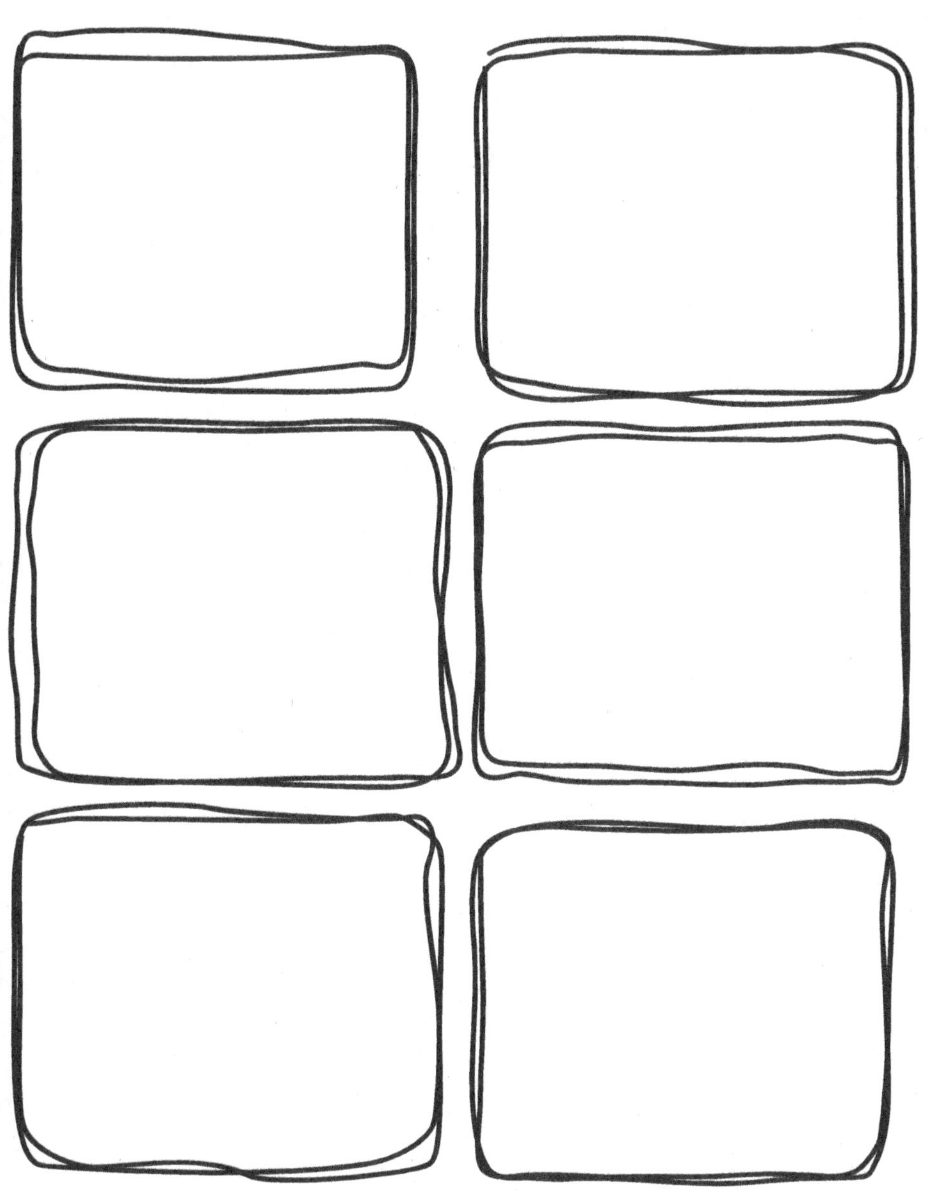

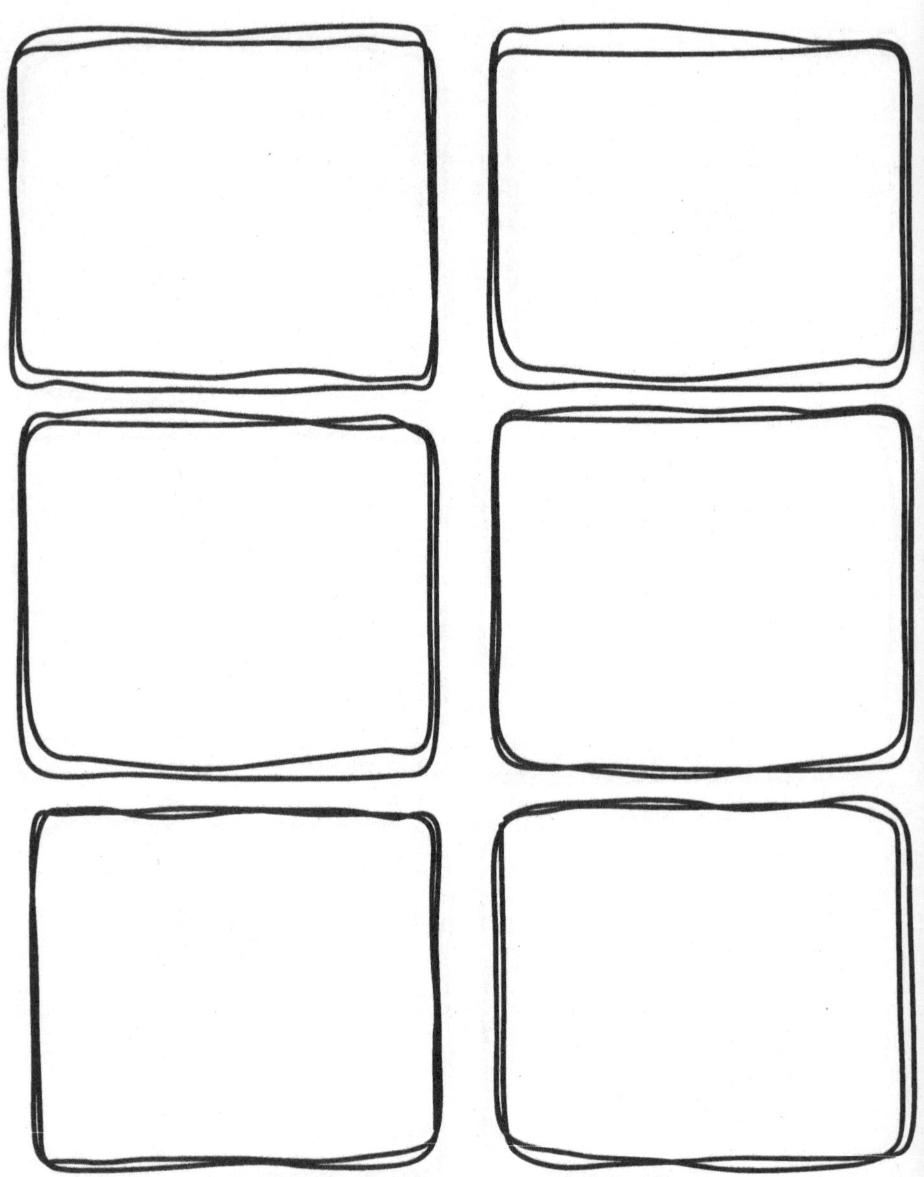

Put a star next to the memories that were most impactful in either a positive or negative way.

What messages about yourself did you internalize from these events?

personal burdens

Every part is burdened, not just exiles. Some of those burdens are personal ones and others are legacy burdens that came from someone else. You will explore some of the burdens that your parts have experienced, or may currently be experiencing. By understanding these burdens, you can help parts know they aren't alone and provide support for them. Even naming and acknowledging burdens can be a source of relief or freedom for parts.

Let's explore some of the personal burdens your parts may be carrying, knowingly or unknowingly. Personal burdens are burdens that have been passed on to you from direct encounters with other people such as family, teachers, authority figures, romantic interests, strangers, or friends, or from traumatizing events. Burdens could be something you experienced directly or witnessed indirectly.

→ ***Circle* any of these personal burdens your parts may have experienced.**

Experiences that left you with personal burdens

Explosive anger	Belittling	Bullying
Verbal abuse	Manipulation	Sarcasm
Passive aggressiveness	Shaming	Guilt tripping
Scapegoating	Domestic violence	Abuse
Violence	Trauma	Toxic relationships
Crime victim	Neglect	Injury
Gaslighting	Humiliation	Addictions
Mental illness	Rejection	Microaggressions

Add any personal burdens your parts have experienced that are not on the list.

How do you feel toward the parts that are holding these burdens?

If you can open your heart to them, then take some time right now to connect with those parts and tell them how you feel.

cultural & legacy burdens

In addition to personal burdens, we take in extreme beliefs and emotions that are from traumas experienced by our ethnic group, perhaps decades or even centuries ago. For example, many Black people in the US carry the pain of their ancestors from years of slavery, and many Jews carry terror and "never again" beliefs from the Holocaust. In addition, there are burdens floating around in the country in which you were raised that some parts of you couldn't help but absorb (even if, like racism for example, those beliefs are abhorrent to you). We call those *cultural legacy burdens*.

Let's identify some cultural and legacy burdens your parts may have experienced or may be experiencing. Pay attention to changes in your body. If you need to pause or skip this exercise you can. Honor your inner system.

Here is a list of some burdens commonly associated with cultural and legacy burdens (this is not an exhaustive list).

↗ *Circle* any of the burdens that resonate with your lived experience.

Cultural & Legacy Burdens

Don't trust anyone	Don't rock the boat	Don't talk about feelings
You need to have it all together	Stay silent about abuse	Vulnerability is weakness
Shame about sexuality	Don't ask for help	Shame about cultural identity
Toxic masculinity	Unhealthy food habits	Unhealthy financial habits
Entitlement/privilege	Poverty	Racism
Sexism	Classism	Discrimination
Homophobia	Xenophobia	Patriarchy
White supremacy	White fragility	White savior complex
Cultural assimilation	Not being ____ enough	Survival guilt
Gentrification	Incarceration	Racial profiling
Ignorance	Collective trauma	War/violence
Political oppression	Pollution	Disease/famine

Were there other cultural burdens your parts have experienced?

What cultural or legacy burdens from the list feel the heaviest for you?

Find a part that carries such a burden and ask: At what age did you start carrying those burdens?

How do you feel toward those parts who were forced to carry those burdens so young?

If you feel compassion, pause and take a moment to express those feelings to those parts.

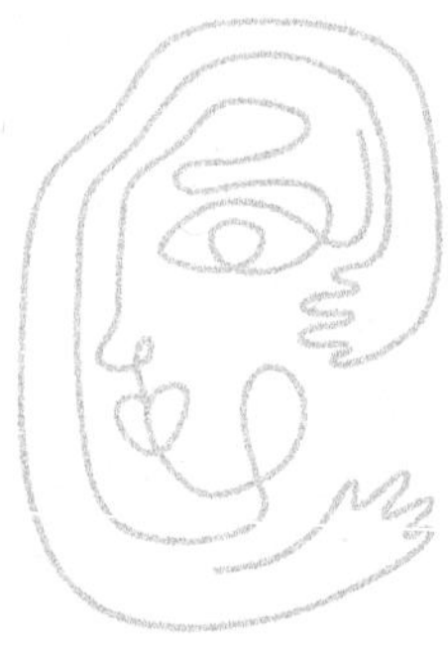

Going Inside Notice how your parts are responding to the topic of cultural and legacy burdens. What emotions are you feeling? Anger? Fear? Sadness? Let your parts know that you are here with them and that whatever they are feeling is okay.

heirlooms

Acknowledging burdens can be an important step to healing them, but appreciating the gifts that we receive from individuals, culture, and family legacy can also be part of the healing process. These gifts are like heirlooms handed down from ancestors. They might be positive character traits like generosity that your parts learned from a family member, or inner resources like resilience that were developed through social trauma.

What are some personal, cultural, and legacy gifts you've received?

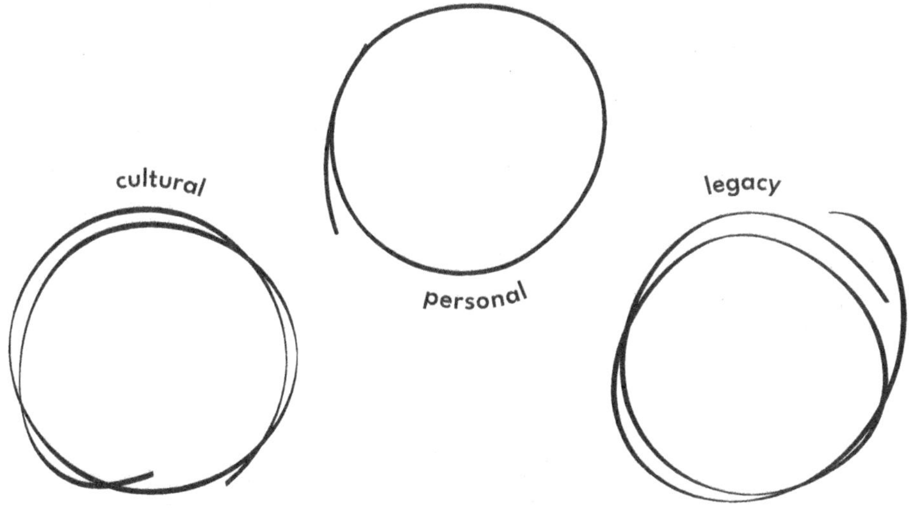

unburdening

Parts carry burdens and parts can be unburdened. While unburdening exiles is beyond the scope of this workbook, and should only be done with a licensed IFS professional, you may have already experienced some relief simply by befriending and connecting with your parts. If you have interest in unburdening your exiles, contact a licensed IFS professional to guide you through the process. In this exercise, you will imagine what it might be like if you didn't have to carry the burdens any longer.

In the space below, write down how you imagine you'd feel if your inner exiles no longer had to carry their burdens.

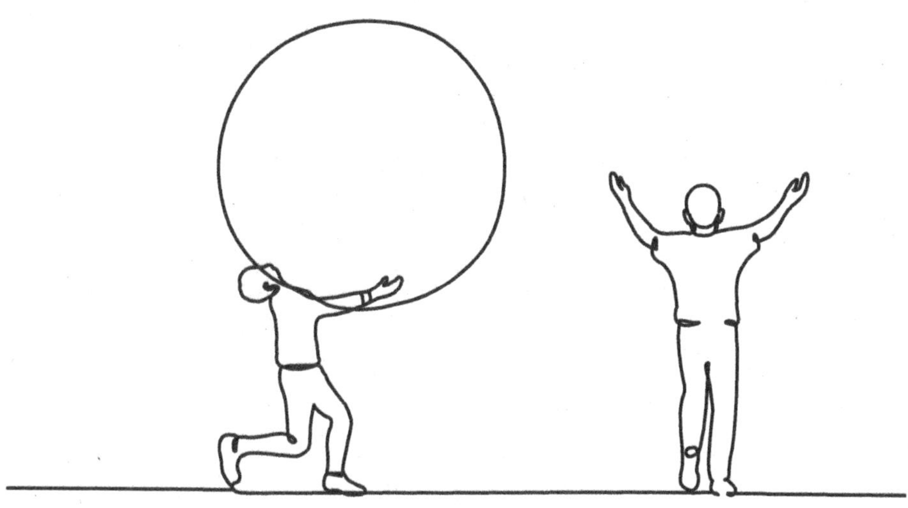

Which burdens are you most interested in unburdening?

Which workbook exercises or IFS practices helped you feel the most relief or freedom?

holding discomfort

Your inner exiles hold your deepest sadness, fear, or sense of worthlessness. When you're in Self, you can sit with parts in their sadness without it deregulating your entire system. This doesn't mean it will be easy, or that you won't have protectors jump back in to distract or derail you. They surely will. But at least now you know how to connect to those parts and ask them to step back.

As you practice connecting with Self and get more comfortable with all your emotions and parts, you will be able to hold discomfort and sit with your parts in their sadness without totally blending with them. That is, you'll be able to *be with* them without *becoming* them. This will help them know that they are not alone anymore, and that someone else in there cares and wants to help them.

You might even want to apologize to them for letting other parts influence you to lock them away. This will help your parts trust you and feel less alone, and experience healing as they feel your Self-energy and compassion.

In this exercise, you'll have the opportunity to hold discomfort by sitting with your exiles' sadness and grieving together.

For the next few minutes, give your parts permission to be sad.

What are some situations in your life, either from the past or present, that fill you with deep sadness?

What do you usually do when you're sad? Do manager parts try to keep you busy so you don't have time to feel? Do firefighters swoop in to rescue you from pain with mind-numbing activities?

Imagine you're sitting in a circle with your parts. Tell them all, "It's okay to be sad." Let them know you can handle their emotions. You may even feel led to apologize for not being able to hold their emotions before now.

How do your parts respond to hearing these things from you?

Ask them if there is anything they want to tell you or show you. Write it down if you'd like.

Do they have any unresolved grief?

Give them some space to grieve with you over those moments. You may want to play some reflective music, sad songs, or blues music to help your parts get in touch with their sadness.

Close your eyes if you'd like and take five to ten minutes to hold the discomfort and sit with your parts in their sadness. When you're done, you can open your eyes and continue.

What was this exercise like for you? What insights did you gain?

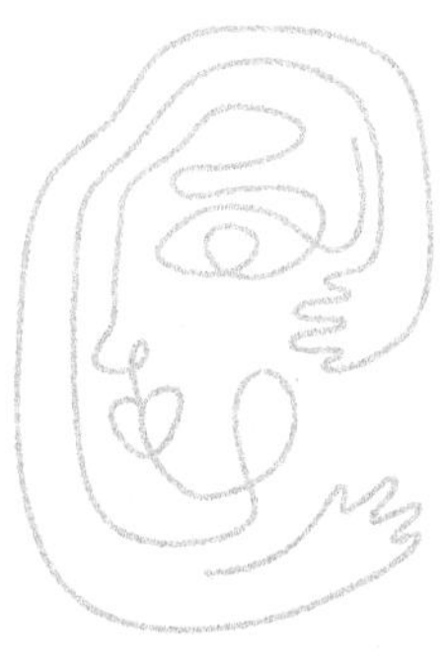

Going Inside You might want to pause here. Take a minute to sit with any parts that are coming up. Let them know they are not alone. Listen to anything they are telling you.

self-portrait

When you focus on your inner exiles, what do you see? Seeing your exiles can be a way to connect with your parts and discover more about them. You may gain insight into their age, where they are, or how they are feeling. Some people, however, don't see anything when they focus inside, and instead hear parts' voices or feel their energy, so don't despair if that's your experience. Parts may not even appear as human, so stay open to whatever comes to you.

In this exercise, you will have a chance to visualize your exiles, your younger parts.

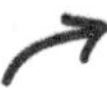

If you can see an exile, draw a picture of it using crayons, markers, or colored pencils. You can use the questions below to guide you:

- What do they look like?
- How old are they?
- Are they wearing anything?
- What emotions or facial expressions do they have?
- What items, if any, are they holding?
- Where are they? Are there any other people in the scene?

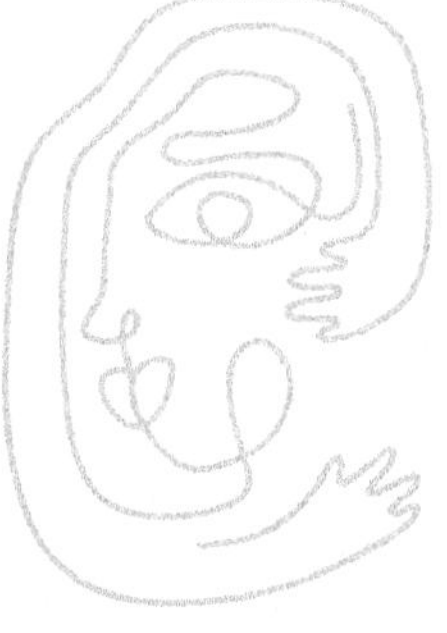

Going Inside Take a moment to go inside and see how your exiled part feels about your drawing. Do they like it? Do they feel seen? Is there anything they would add?

exile meditation

This is a meditation to get to know your exiled parts. You may or may not be able to fully connect with your exiles if you haven't worked enough yet with your protectors. Some people work for years with their protective system before they are allowed access to their exiles. If you push too hard too fast, your protectors may come back even stronger. Trust your system to let you know when it's ready. If it feels like too much for your parts, you can stop at any point. You can always come back to this meditation when your parts feel ready. An audio recording of this practice is available at:

soundstrue.com/the-ifs-workbook-bonus

Sit in a comfortable chair or even lie down on a couch.

Close your eyes.

Notice any protector parts that might come up.

Ask them if they would be willing to step back for a few moments. Invite them to watch.

Try to get in touch with your exiles, the vulnerable, young parts of you.

Where do you feel the exile in your body?

How close or far are they from you?

How old are they?

What do they want you to know about them?
What messages or fears do they have?

How do you feel toward them?

If you're feeling compassion, then let them know.
If you're struggling to feel compassion for the part, just listen to see if they have anything else they want you to know about them.

Try to find something you love or appreciate about this exile and speak those words to them.

How does it feel for them to hear how you feel?

How old do they think you are? If they think you are younger than you are, update them on your age and what you are doing now.

Ask this part what it wants or needs from you. Maybe they want to be held, to hear assurance from you that they are loved, or some other gesture.

If you're feeling enough Self-energy, send compassion to this part.

Sit with them for a while. Just enjoy being together.

Ask them if you can check back in with them.

If they are open, make a specific plan to check in on your exile part later this week.

When you're ready, open your eyes.

reparenting your parts

Healing happens for your younger parts when you're able to show them love and compassion from your Self-energy. The Self can provide your parts the love you may have wanted as a child but didn't receive. Now that you're aware of your Self and your parts, you can reparent your parts. You can show them the tenderness and care they are longing for. This can take time. To do this, you need to be connected to your Self. Remember, the best way to know if you're being Self-led is if you're feeling the 8 Cs (Calm, Clarity, Confidence, Curiosity, Connectedness, Creativity, Compassion, and Courage).

In this exercise, you will practice reparenting your parts.

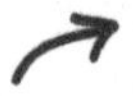

Fill in the answers for each of the questions from your conversations with your exiles.

Which parenting styles do your inner exiles/younger parts prefer?

What attributes of Self do your parts find most nurturing?

How does your inner exile best receive love?

How can you provide that for them?

What kind of reassurance or affirmation does your inner exile want?

How can you provide that for them?

Set up a regular time to connect with your exiled parts to show them love in the way they best receive it.

an adventure with an inner exile

Your inner exiles are often younger parts of you. They will probably like things that you liked as a child and might still enjoy those things. When you feel nostalgia, it might be because your exiles, or other younger parts, are carrying feelings related to those memories. A time, a place, an antique item, or a toy may awaken your exiles' memories or emotions. As you get to know them, you can take them on imaginary or real-life adventures, where they can be kids again and they can spend time with you. The more you bring your exiles close to your Self, the deeper the connection will be and the more healing they can experience. It's also important to remember that the closer they get to you, the more access you have to their wonderful qualities that you had been cut off from.

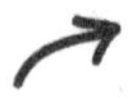

In this exercise, you will go on an adventure with your inner exile. Ask that part:

What place, real or imagined, would they like to go?

Why is this place meaningful to them?

What do they want to bring with them?

What activities do they want to do with you?

Set aside some time to go with your inner exile on this adventure in your inner world and reflect on it below.

What was this like for them?

What was it like for you?

If it's a real place, you might want to plan a trip to the actual place. If it's an imaginary place, set up a time in the future where you can take them again in your mind.

part five

accessing your unlimited self-leadership

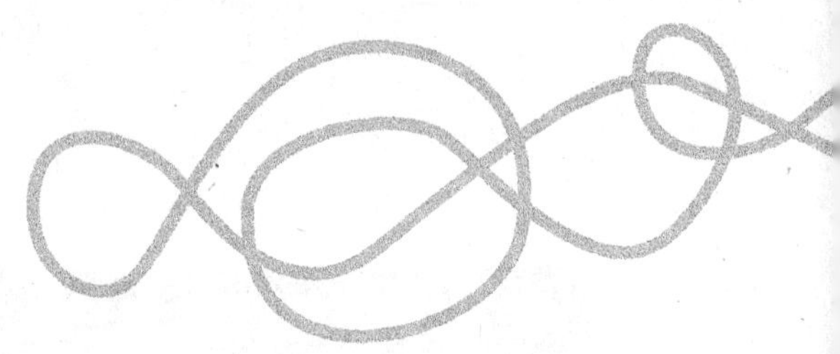

Let's stop and take a moment to appreciate how far you've come. In Part Four, you went to some deep places. You spent time with your inner exiles. You've identified some of the burdens your parts are carrying from family, culture, and society. You have learned to reparent and partner with your parts so you can be more integrated. You've explored your Self, your protectors, and your exiles. You've learned to go inside, and extended compassion and healing to your parts. Well done.

In Part Five, you will find additional tools and resources to deepen your Self-leadership and incorporate the qualities of Self into all aspects of your life. When you are aware of and attuned to your parts, and they are willing to separate from you a bit, you are able to be Self-led. Self-leadership happens when your Self takes the lead. It's possible to move in and out of Self-leadership as parts are dynamic and situations can cause activation. Working with parts on an ongoing basis is necessary. As you develop Self-leadership in your inner system, you'll be able to bring those same qualities of Self into your outer world.

Being Self-led is a process and a daily practice. Look for ways to incorporate these practices into your everyday life.

By practicing Self-leadership, you are making a difference in your life, in your work, and in the world.

self-leadership assessment

Rate yourself on a scale of 1 to 10 (1 = low Self and 10 = high Self) in each of the following categories.

Mark where you are on the spectrum and write the date. You can revisit this assessment regularly to see what progress you've made in these areas.

1. **Self-awareness** I am aware of my parts and I am able to speak for them.

   1 2 3 4 5 6 7 8 9 10

2. **Self-care** I listen and respond to the needs of my parts with appropriate care and action.

   1 2 3 4 5 6 7 8 9 10

3. **Self-healing** I am connected to my parts and have regular times to touch base and extend appreciation and compassion to them.

   1 2 3 4 5 6 7 8 9 10

4. **Self-energy** I am able to maintain Self-energy even when my parts are activated.

1 2 3 4 5 6 7 8 9 10

5. **Self-talk** I talk positively to myself and to my parts.

1 2 3 4 5 6 7 8 9 10

6. **Self-love** I feel genuine love for myself and my parts and express that love daily.

1 2 3 4 5 6 7 8 9 10

7. **Self-leadership** I am able to lead from my Self at most times.

1 2 3 4 5 6 7 8 9 10

Tally your numbers. Enter the numbers from the evaluation below:

1. ___ 2. ___ 3. ___ 4. ___ 5. ___ 6. ___ 7. ___

Total: ___

Divide that number by 7.

Your average Self-leadership score:

1–4 — Low Self-leadership

5–7 — Medium Self-leadership

8–10 — High Self-leadership

Don't be discouraged if your Self-leadership isn't high. Keep practicing what you've learned. Work with your parts and come back every few weeks to see if your score changes.

courage: a meditation

True courage is one of the most difficult qualities of the Self to access. This meditation will help you learn to embody courage and other qualities of the Self. Remember, these attributes are always there inside you. With practice, you can access this Self-energy anytime, anywhere. An audio recording of this practice is available at:

soundstrue.com/the-ifs-workbook-bonus

Take some deep breaths.

Think of a time in your life when you felt a lot of courage.

Maybe it was a time when you had the courage to act or speak about something scary.

Was there a time when you had the courage to do something that a lot of your parts were afraid to do?

Take some time to scan through your past. Look at different points, until you find the time that feels right.

When you find that courageous version of you, put that person in a room by themselves and look at that person through a window.

See how you feel toward that earlier version of you who held such courage, clarity, and strength. See how your parts react to that person. See if they'd be willing to embody that quality again, to be that you and enter into that space even though circumstances are different now.

If they're not willing, that's okay. You can just explore their fears about what would happen if you embodied that quality of Self even for a little while.

But if they are willing, then go ahead and enter the room, and step into that person's body and feel that courage in your body now. Just notice what it feels like again. See how your parts react to your being in that courageous state again.

When the time feels right, begin to shift your focus back to the outside world, but see how possible it is to hold this courageous, clear, strong state even as you come back. Even as you open your eyes.

becoming a self-led leader

The IFS model can help you develop Self-leadership so you can heal your parts and become more Self-led in your home, work, and community.

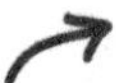

Select one or two ideas from each list to apply to your everyday life. You can also add your own ideas.

In Your Home

- Model speaking for parts with your family.
- Get curious about your parts and those of your family.
- Reparent your own parts so you can better parent your children.
- Teach your kids to use parts language.

In Your Professional Life

- Model speaking for parts with your coworkers.
- When you're activated, check in with your parts.
- When a colleague is in a protector, try to imagine the exile that's likely driving it.

In Your Community

- Show compassion for other people's parts.
- Share what you're learning about your parts with your friend groups.
- Go through this workbook with a small group.
- Organize others to understand and take action around specific cultural burdens that are impacting your community.

end of day inventory

This practice can help you stay attuned to your inner system from day to day. At the end of each day, consider doing an inventory of your parts.

Write down which parts showed up. When were you Self-led? When were you not?

Parts Inventory

Parts that showed up today:

When did I act Self-led?

When was I not Self-led?

outward bound

It may seem counterintuitive, but doing inner work can actually move you to engage the outer world. When you become more Self-led, you become less ego-driven, less focused on your own inner struggles, and you develop more altruistic characteristics.

With the Clarity attribute of Self, you see the injustice and suffering in the world and have more Compassion. You will often become more active to change things in big and small ways.

What parts of you like the thought of engaging the world with more Compassion?

What stops you from showing Compassion?

How might being Self-led change the way you engage the outside world?

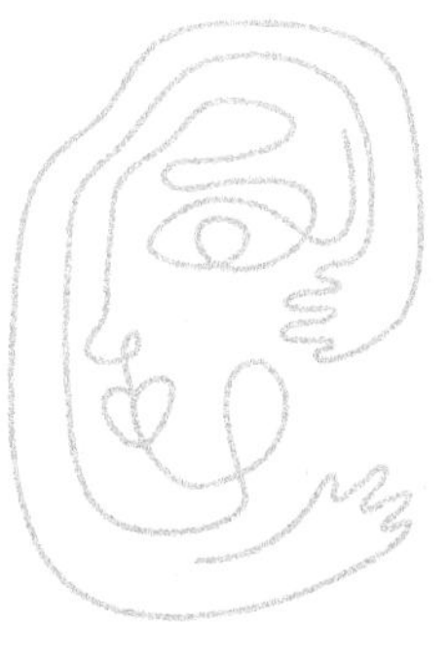

Going Inside Notice any parts that might be fearful or reluctant to extend Compassion to others. Take some time to work with those parts. Find, Focus, and Flesh Out what those protectors are feeling. If you have enough Curiosity, BeFriend those parts and extend Compassion to them. Appreciate them for how they're wanting to protect you. See if they're willing to trust you to take the lead. If not, ask them why not.

a playlist for your parts

Parts like being acknowledged and appreciated. One way to do this is to make a playlist for your parts. Choose a song that represents each part and make a playlist that you can listen to and celebrate each part.

Use the space here to write down the names of your parts on the left side and a song that reflects each part on the right side.

Select one song for each part, then create the playlist on your favorite listening device to enjoy with all your parts.

Part	Song

accessing self-energy

It's not always easy to access Self-energy. Especially when parts are activated. A simple yet effective exercise is to find those things in your everyday life that naturally bring Self-energy into your system. This is something you can explore.

What helps you tap into your Self-energy? What helps you separate from activated thoughts and emotions and be more Self-led?

Some activities might include:

- Going for a walk in your neighborhood
- Watching a sunrise or sunset
- Being in or around nature
- Looking out at a body of water
- Watching the activity at a bird feeder
- Playing with pets
- Spending time with children or grandchildren
- Rubbing your heart with your hand
- Listening to music
- Getting away from activating people

What activities in your everyday life bring Self-energy into your system?

IFS Tip

Start to explore the areas or moments in your life where you naturally feel Self-energy and inner peace. If possible, make these things part of your daily life. Return to them when your body is activated in order to be a little less activated. Find what works for you to make Self-energy more available in your system.

self-care checklist

Self-care involves attending to your parts. When parts are neglected or ignored, they can act out in ways you least expect or desire. By checking in with your parts, you can assure the managers, firefighters, and exiles that they are not alone and that you are there to support them if they get activated.

→ **Look at the following Self-care activities and see which ones appeal to your parts.**

Think of ways you can incorporate IFS into these Self-care activities. Sometimes there are real constraints that may prevent you from doing some of them, but sometimes there are parts that are preventing Self-care that you can work with.

- Speak for your parts to loved ones about what your parts need from them or want them to know
- Do something creative
- Go outside in nature
- Take a nap in the middle of the day
- Get a massage
- Take a vacation
- Go on a date with yourself
- Read a book for fun
- Cook your favorite meal
- Play like a child
- Dance
- Try something new
- Do something adventurous
- Connect with friends
- Do something spontaneous
- Make love
- Smell flowers
- Eat your favorite sweet treat
- Prioritize your own joy

Are there other Self-care practices you would add to the list?

How might you incorporate parts work into these activities?

If it's been a while since you've done some of these Self-care practices, make a plan to do three Self-care activities this week.

This week I will do the following three things:

1. ______

2. ______

3. ______

self-love

Healing happens when you're able to love your parts, all of them. This is the epitome of Self-love. There are other techniques that encourage you to have love or compassion for many parts, but not those that seem irritating, destructive, or dangerous. IFS is different in this way.

In this exercise, you will explore ways to love yourself. Fill in other ways you can show love to yourself.

- Give yourself a hug

- Remind yourself there are no bad parts

- Spend time listening to your parts, even the ones that, on initial examination, seem to have no redeeming value

- Once you learn where your parts are stuck in time, and how they are trying to protect, extend appreciation and love to them too

a picture is worth a thousand words

It's possible to recognize parts from pictures. You can look at old pictures of yourself to see what parts you notice. You might see a people-pleasing part at a birthday party or a lonely part at a family event. It can be helpful to revisit moments in time to learn what parts may have been in the driver's seat.

For this exercise, you will need to get some old pictures or photo albums. See if you can identify parts from the pictures. Write down any insights you have.

Picture:

Date:

Part:

Insights:

Picture:

Date:

Part:

Insights:

Picture:

Date:

Part:

Insights:

Picture:

Date:

Part:

Insights:

being your own hope merchant

A hope merchant is someone who offers the possibility of change for those in hopeless situations. You may discover parts that believe or think there's no reason or possibility to change. They may have trouble trusting your Self-leadership or doubt anyone else could run things as well as they can. When you are connected to Self, you are able to become a hope merchant for your parts by letting them know that change and healing are truly possible.

In this exercise, you'll have an opportunity to come up with hope merchant statements for your parts.

Think back to your protector and exile fears. What are the messages they are most desperate to hear from you? What sincere feelings and hopes can you share with them? Make sure you connect with your Self-energy because hope merchant messages flow naturally from Self.

In the spaces below, write four or five messages you want your parts to trust.

Example: *I love you for who you are, not for what you do or don't do.*

Take some time to remind your parts of these truths about you.

IFS Tip

Write your truths about yourself down on Post-it notes and place them by your mirror or desk where you can see them and be reminded.

IFS practices for everyday life

Let's review some of the experiential and embodied practices you've learned throughout this workbook.

Going inside	Getting to know your managers and firefighters
Connecting with Self	Showing appreciation to parts
Finding parts	Listening to exile fears
Befriending parts	Holding discomfort
Using parts language	Identifying burdens
Mapping your parts	Reparenting your younger parts
Locating parts in your body	Being Self-led
Doing a one-minute daily check-in	Practicing Self-love
Doing a daily parts inventory	Being a hope merchant for your parts

What practices in this workbook have been the most impactful for you and your parts?

What practices do you need to spend more time developing?

What practices would you like to incorporate into your everyday life?

trailheads for future exploration

When you're hiking, you'll find the head of a trail. If you follow that trail, it might take you to a shimmering lake or cascading waterfall. There are also trailheads inside of you. When you focus on parts, you might become aware of a trail that you want to explore in the future. You may have experienced this as you've gone through the workbook.

In this exercise, you'll identify some trailheads within you for future exploration so you can continue the work you started.

You can also take suggestions from this list for how to identify trailheads:

- Notice which parts come up in certain places, with certain people, and when you're performing different roles.
- Notice what emotions come up as you explore different parts.

- Notice what triggers your anger. Is there sadness underneath? Is there fear of being taken advantage of? Spend time exploring these triggers.
- Notice what activates your deepest sadness. Chances are that's where you'll find your exiles.
- Burdens can be personal, cultural, or legacy burdens. Explore these burdens with an IFS counselor or group.
- What parts are you most interested in exploring further? Managers, firefighters, or exiles? Spend time with parts you are least familiar with or have the hardest time loving.
- How can you tell whether you are in Self or not? What markers do you use to check? Some suggestions: Is my heart open right now? Do I have a big agenda? Am I calm? Confident? Clear? How much am I in my body?
- Notice when you are in Self and when you are not in Self in any given situation. What helps you stay in Self? What takes you out of Self? What helps you return once you've been activated? Use these trailheads for further exploration.

Future Trailheads:

a closing letter from Dick

Dear Friend,

Congratulations on completing this workbook!

It is my hope that you have gotten to know some of your parts, discovered your Self, and experienced positive shifts in the way you relate with yourself. I hope this work has allowed you to bring more compassion and love to your parts and that this has created more Self-compassion and healing inside.

Hopefully, your parts are learning to trust that they don't have to take over like they used to. They can trust you to lead. As you make this work part of your everyday life, you will relate from Self to others more and more, and feel more harmonious inside.

Remember, this is a lifelong practice. You're going to put some things in place, and you may do them for a little while, and then life is going to get in the way. It's natural to have times when you're going to stop doing them. That's okay. That's to be expected. Once you've done this work though, it's like riding a bike. You can always come back to it. You may need to just revisit some of the exercises or you may want to redo the whole workbook. This is a tool to return to again and again.

As I said at the outset, this is a journey. Follow the trailheads. Explore your inner terrain. And most importantly, enjoy the ride!

Congratulations again!

A Merchant of Hope,

Dick Schwartz

IFS resources

Richard C. Schwartz, *Introduction to Internal Family Systems* (Vermilion, 2023).

—, *You Are the One You've Been Waiting For: Applying Internal Family Systems to Intimate Relationships* (Vermilion, 2023).

—, *No Bad Parts: Healing Trauma and Restoring Wholeness with the Internal Family Systems Model* (Vermilion, 2023).

—, *Greater Than the Sum of Our Parts: Discovering Your True Self Through Internal Family Systems Therapy* (Sounds True, 2018).

For information on IFS Institute's growing number of courses or to find an IFS practitioner, visit ifs-institute.com.

If you're in crisis you may try the following services for assistance.

US Base: Dial 9-8-8 for the Suicide & Crisis Lifeline

For US or International support visit: findahelpline.com

*Note: IFS Institute is not affiliated with these support lines.

acknowledgments

This IFS journey is now forty years old. The list of people who have contributed to its development is extremely long and I have tried to thank them elsewhere. For this book, I want to particularly thank our IFS staff and trainers, all of whom work so hard to bring IFS to the world, including a small group who supported the research and reviewing of this material. I feel blessed to have so many talented people helping me bring IFS to you.

I'm also extremely grateful to Tami Simon and all of her staff at Sounds True for their wonderful support on this and my other books.

about the author

Richard C. Schwartz, PhD, is the creator of Internal Family Systems, a highly effective, evidence-based therapeutic model that de-pathologizes the multipart personality. His IFS Institute offers training for professionals and the general public. Formerly an associate professor in the Department of Psychiatry at the University of Illinois at Chicago and later at Northwestern University, he is currently on the faculty of Harvard Medical School. He is a sought-after presenter and the author of several books, including *No Bad Parts*, *You Are the One You've Been Waiting For*, and *Introduction to Internal Family Systems*. For more, visit ifs-institute.com.